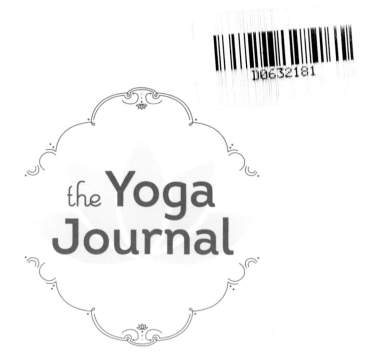

the Yoga Journal

CHRONICLE BOOKS
SAN FRANCISCO

ISBN: 978-1-4521-3916-6

Manufactured in China

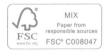

FSC
www.fsc.org

MIX
Paper from
responsible sources
FSC® C008047

Designed by Mia Johnson

The information, practices, and poses in this book are not
offered as medical advice or suggested as treatment
for any condition that might require medical attention.
To avoid injury, practice yoga with a skilled instructor and
consult a health professional to determine your body's
needs and limitations. The writer and publisher hereby
disclaim any liability from injuries resulting from following
any recommendation in this book.

10 9 8 7 6 5 4 3 2 1

Chronicle Books LLC
680 Second Street
San Francisco, California 94107
www.chroniclebooks.com

Contents

About This Journal 5

Before You Begin: My Yoga Profile 6

At-A-Glance Records:

    Yoga Friends and Family 8

    Yoga Studio Log 10

    Yoga Instructor Log 12

    One-Year Practice Log 16

    My Dedication Log 18

    My Yoga Soundtrack 20

    My Collection of Yoga Wisdom 22

    Yoga Around the World 24

    Yoga Gear to Get 28

    Yoga Festivals and Events to Check Out 29

    Yoga Books to Read 30

    Yoga Websites to Visit 31

    General Health Tracker: Symptoms 32

    General Health Tracker: Treatments 34

    General Health Tracker: Medications
    and Nutritional Supplements 36

    For Yoga Moms: My Prenatal Practice 38

    For Yoga Moms: My Postnatal Practice 40

    My Goals 42

Yoga Session Journal 43

Yoga Reference Guide 135

    A Brief History of Yoga 136

    The Branches of Yoga 138

    Yoga Styles 139

    Yoga Philosophy 144

    Illustrated Yoga Pose Directory 148

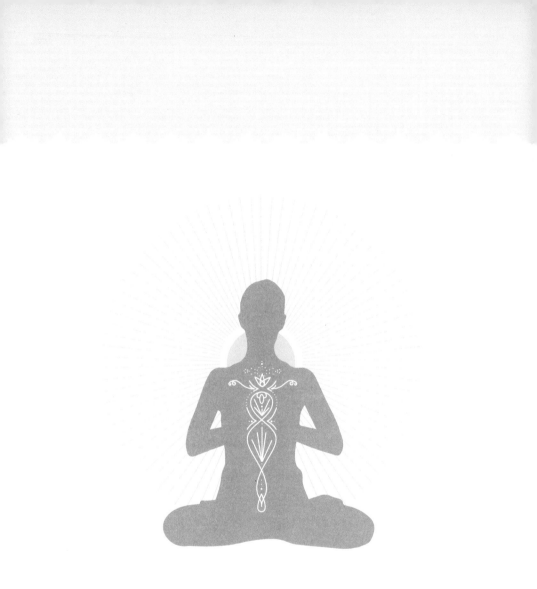

About This Journal

Self-study is an important part of any yoga practice. Get to know your inner yogi by recording your experiences in the pages of this journal. Whether you have attended only five classes or five hundred; whether you do yoga for health and healing or just for fun; and whether you are committed to one style of yoga or enjoy exploring them all, *The Yoga Journal* will take you deeper into your practice and lead you to enriching self-discoveries, on and off the mat.

Start by turning this page and completing "My Yoga Profile." Then, over time, fill out the at-a-glance records and checklists that address key aspects of your practice, from setting goals and monitoring progress to keeping track of favorite instructors and studios. The next time you do yoga, turn to one of the guided journal entries in the second half of the book and log the details of that session. With space for recording forty-five individual sessions, this journal invites you to see how truly dynamic a yoga practice can be. After all, no two yoga sessions are alike. Each is unique, varying not only in pose sequencing but also in the day-to-day fluctuations of your moods, energy levels, and interests.

Indeed, your yoga practice is a living, ever-evolving entity—just like you. Watch it flourish in these pages as you grow stronger, more balanced, and more present in your daily life.

Namaste.

My Yoga Profile

Complete this profile and share it with your yoga instructors and health coaches who can help you create a customized yoga practice that best meets your needs.

NAME .... TODAY'S DATE .... / .... / ....

CONTACT INFORMATION ....

....

AGE .... WHEN DID YOU FIRST GIVE YOGA A TRY? ....

                                                                                    (MONTH)   (YEAR)

DESCRIBE YOUR FIRST IMPRESSIONS OF YOGA ....

....

....

NUMBER OF CLASSES YOU'VE TAKEN IN THE PAST THREE YEARS

☐ 5 OR LESS   ☐ 6-20   ☐ 21-40   ☐ MORE THAN 40

YOUR CURRENT SKILL LEVEL

☐ FIRST-TIMER   ☐ BEGINNER   ☐ ADVANCED BEGINNER   ☐ EARLY INTERMEDIATE   ☐ INTERMEDIATE

☐ ADVANCED INTERMEDIATE   ☐ ADVANCED   ☐ TEACHER-IN-TRAINING   ☐ INSTRUCTOR

WHICH YOGA STYLES HAVE YOU TRIED?

☐ ANUSARA   ☐ ASHTANGA   ☐ BIKRAM   ☐ IYENGAR   ☐ JIVAMUKTI

☐ KRIPALU   ☐ KUNDALINI   ☐ POWER   ☐ RESTORATIVE   ☐ OTHER: ....

WHAT BENEFITS ARE YOU SEEKING IN YOUR YOGA PRACTICE? (CHECK ALL THAT APPLY.)

☐ BODY SCULPTING   ☐ PHYSICAL FITNESS   ☐ FLEXIBILITY   ☐ INCREASED STRENGTH   ☐ IMPROVED BALANCE

☐ STRESS REDUCTION   ☐ ENHANCED SLEEP   ☐ GENERAL HEALTH AND WELL-BEING   ☐ SPIRITUAL ENRICHMENT

☐ OTHER ....   ☐ OTHER ....   ☐ OTHER ....

EMERGENCY CONTACT

NAME .... RELATIONSHIP ....

CONTACT INFORMATION ....

....

Past and current injuries and/or health conditions:

TO RECORD ADDITIONAL INJURIES AND CONDITIONS, TURN TO THE HEALTH TRACKER (PAGES 32-37).

DESCRIBE INJURY/CONDITION ....

.... WHEN DID THE INJURY OCCUR? ....

                                                                     (MONTH)   (YEAR)

HAVE YOU COMPLETELY RECOVERED? ☐ YES ☐ NO

IF YES, WHEN WAS RECOVERY COMPLETE? ....

                                        (MONTH)   (YEAR)

DESCRIBE INJURY/CONDITION ....

.... WHEN DID THE INJURY OCCUR? ....

                                        (MONTH)   (YEAR)

HAVE YOU COMPLETELY RECOVERED? ☐ YES ☐ NO

IF YES, WHEN WAS RECOVERY COMPLETE? ....

                                        (MONTH)   (YEAR)

DESCRIBE INJURY/CONDITION ....

.... WHEN DID THE INJURY OCCUR? ....

                                        (MONTH)   (YEAR)

HAVE YOU COMPLETELY RECOVERED? ☐ YES ☐ NO

IF YES, WHEN WAS RECOVERY COMPLETE? ....

                                        (MONTH)   (YEAR)

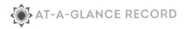

Yoga Friends and Family

Log contact information here to build relationships and stay in touch
with your growing yoga community.

NAME

TEL

EMAIL

NOTES

NAME

TEL

EMAIL

NOTES

NAME

TEL

EMAIL

NOTES

NAME

TEL

EMAIL

NOTES

NAME

TEL

EMAIL

NOTES

NAME

TEL

EMAIL

NOTES

NAME

TEL

EMAIL

NOTES

NAME

TEL

EMAIL

NOTES

NAME

TEL

EMAIL

NOTES

NAME

TEL

EMAIL

NOTES

NAME

TEL

EMAIL

NOTES

NAME

TEL

EMAIL

NOTES

NAME

TEL

EMAIL

NOTES

NAME

TEL

EMAIL

NOTES

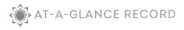
Yoga Studio Log

Record the local studios you've visited, and those you want to visit, to create a helpful log of the yoga centers in your area.

STUDIO NAME

LOCATION

PRIMARY YOGA STYLE

NOTEWORTHY INSTRUCTOR(S)

☐ VISITED ON THESE DATES: OR ☐ HAVEN'T BEEN/WANT TO GO

STUDIO NAME

LOCATION

PRIMARY YOGA STYLE

NOTEWORTHY INSTRUCTOR(S)

☐ VISITED ON THESE DATES: OR ☐ HAVEN'T BEEN/WANT TO GO

STUDIO NAME

LOCATION

PRIMARY YOGA STYLE

NOTEWORTHY INSTRUCTOR(S)

☐ VISITED ON THESE DATES: OR ☐ HAVEN'T BEEN/WANT TO GO

STUDIO NAME

LOCATION

PRIMARY YOGA STYLE

NOTEWORTHY INSTRUCTOR(S)

☐ VISITED ON THESE DATES: OR ☐ HAVEN'T BEEN/WANT TO GO

STUDIO NAME

LOCATION

PRIMARY YOGA STYLE

NOTEWORTHY INSTRUCTOR(S)

☐ VISITED ON THESE DATES: OR ☐ HAVEN'T BEEN/WANT TO GO

STUDIO NAME

LOCATION

PRIMARY YOGA STYLE

NOTEWORTHY INSTRUCTOR(S)

☐ VISITED ON THESE DATES:

OR

☐ HAVEN'T BEEN/WANT TO GO

STUDIO NAME

LOCATION

PRIMARY YOGA STYLE

NOTEWORTHY INSTRUCTOR(S)

☐ VISITED ON THESE DATES:

OR

☐ HAVEN'T BEEN/WANT TO GO

STUDIO NAME

LOCATION

PRIMARY YOGA STYLE

NOTEWORTHY INSTRUCTOR(S)

☐ VISITED ON THESE DATES:

OR

☐ HAVEN'T BEEN/WANT TO GO

STUDIO NAME

LOCATION

PRIMARY YOGA STYLE

NOTEWORTHY INSTRUCTOR(S)

☐ VISITED ON THESE DATES:

OR

☐ HAVEN'T BEEN/WANT TO GO

STUDIO NAME

LOCATION

PRIMARY YOGA STYLE

NOTEWORTHY INSTRUCTOR(S)

☐ VISITED ON THESE DATES:

OR

☐ HAVEN'T BEEN/WANT TO GO

STUDIO NAME

LOCATION

PRIMARY YOGA STYLE

NOTEWORTHY INSTRUCTOR(S)

☐ VISITED ON THESE DATES:

OR

☐ HAVEN'T BEEN/WANT TO GO

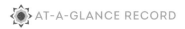

Yoga Instructor Log

Note the characteristics of the instructors you've tried, and explore new instructors throughout your community. Rate each of them according to your personal preferences.

Instructor's name

STUDIO/S WHERE HE/SHE TEACHES

THIS INSTRUCTOR INCORPORATES THE FOLLOWING INTO HIS/HER CLASSES:

☐ INSPIRATIONAL COMMENTARY   ☐ HANDS-ON MODIFICATIONS   ☐ CHANTING   ☐ BREATHING EXERCISES

☐ OTHER:

PACE OF FLOW (CIRCLE ONE):   FAST   MODERATE   SLOW

INSTRUCTOR RATINGS: POSE SEQUENCING: CLARITY OF INSTRUCTION: OVERALL RANKING:
A+ A A- B C D F   A+ A A- B C D F   A+ A A- B C D F

NOTES

Instructor's name

STUDIO/S WHERE HE/SHE TEACHES

THIS INSTRUCTOR INCORPORATES THE FOLLOWING INTO HIS/HER CLASSES:

☐ INSPIRATIONAL COMMENTARY   ☐ HANDS-ON MODIFICATIONS   ☐ CHANTING   ☐ BREATHING EXERCISES

☐ OTHER:

PACE OF FLOW (CIRCLE ONE):   FAST   MODERATE   SLOW

INSTRUCTOR RATINGS: POSE SEQUENCING: CLARITY OF INSTRUCTION: OVERALL RANKING:
A+ A A- B C D F   A+ A A- B C D F   A+ A A- B C D F

NOTES

Instructor's name ....

STUDIO/S WHERE HE/SHE TEACHES ....

THIS INSTRUCTOR INCORPORATES THE FOLLOWING INTO HIS/HER CLASSES:

☐ INSPIRATIONAL COMMENTARY   ☐ HANDS-ON MODIFICATIONS   ☐ CHANTING   ☐ BREATHING EXERCISES

☐ OTHER: ....

PACE OF FLOW (CIRCLE ONE):   FAST   MODERATE   SLOW

INSTRUCTOR RATINGS: POSE SEQUENCING: CLARITY OF INSTRUCTION: OVERALL RANKING:
                          A+ A A- B C D F   A+ A A- B C D F   A+ A A- B C D F

NOTES ....

....

Instructor's name ....

STUDIO/S WHERE HE/SHE TEACHES ....

THIS INSTRUCTOR INCORPORATES THE FOLLOWING INTO HIS/HER CLASSES:

☐ INSPIRATIONAL COMMENTARY   ☐ HANDS-ON MODIFICATIONS   ☐ CHANTING   ☐ BREATHING EXERCISES

☐ OTHER: ....

PACE OF FLOW (CIRCLE ONE):   FAST   MODERATE   SLOW

INSTRUCTOR RATINGS: POSE SEQUENCING: CLARITY OF INSTRUCTION: OVERALL RANKING:
                          A+ A A- B C D F   A+ A A- B C D F   A+ A A- B C D F

NOTES ....

....

Instructor's name ....

STUDIO/S WHERE HE/SHE TEACHES ....

THIS INSTRUCTOR INCORPORATES THE FOLLOWING INTO HIS/HER CLASSES:

☐ INSPIRATIONAL COMMENTARY   ☐ HANDS-ON MODIFICATIONS   ☐ CHANTING   ☐ BREATHING EXERCISES

☐ OTHER: ....

PACE OF FLOW (CIRCLE ONE):   FAST   MODERATE   SLOW

INSTRUCTOR RATINGS: POSE SEQUENCING: CLARITY OF INSTRUCTION: OVERALL RANKING:
                          A+ A A- B C D F   A+ A A- B C D F   A+ A A- B C D F

NOTES ....

....

Instructor's name ....

STUDIO/S WHERE HE/SHE TEACHES ....

THIS INSTRUCTOR INCORPORATES THE FOLLOWING INTO HIS/HER CLASSES:

☐ INSPIRATIONAL COMMENTARY ☐ HANDS-ON MODIFICATIONS ☐ CHANTING ☐ BREATHING EXERCISES

☐ OTHER: ....

PACE OF FLOW (CIRCLE ONE):   FAST   MODERATE   SLOW

INSTRUCTOR RATINGS: POSE SEQUENCING: CLARITY OF INSTRUCTION: OVERALL RANKING:
                            A+ A A- B C D F   A+ A A- B C D F   A+ A A- B C D F

NOTES ....

....

Instructor's name ....

STUDIO/S WHERE HE/SHE TEACHES ....

THIS INSTRUCTOR INCORPORATES THE FOLLOWING INTO HIS/HER CLASSES:

☐ INSPIRATIONAL COMMENTARY ☐ HANDS-ON MODIFICATIONS ☐ CHANTING ☐ BREATHING EXERCISES

☐ OTHER: ....

PACE OF FLOW (CIRCLE ONE):   FAST   MODERATE   SLOW

INSTRUCTOR RATINGS: POSE SEQUENCING: CLARITY OF INSTRUCTION: OVERALL RANKING:
                            A+ A A- B C D F   A+ A A- B C D F   A+ A A- B C D F

NOTES ....

....

Instructor's name ....

STUDIO/S WHERE HE/SHE TEACHES ....

THIS INSTRUCTOR INCORPORATES THE FOLLOWING INTO HIS/HER CLASSES:

☐ INSPIRATIONAL COMMENTARY ☐ HANDS-ON MODIFICATIONS ☐ CHANTING ☐ BREATHING EXERCISES

☐ OTHER: ....

PACE OF FLOW (CIRCLE ONE):   FAST   MODERATE   SLOW

INSTRUCTOR RATINGS: POSE SEQUENCING: CLARITY OF INSTRUCTION: OVERALL RANKING:
                            A+ A A- B C D F   A+ A A- B C D F   A+ A A- B C D F

NOTES ....

....

Instructor's name ....

STUDIO/S WHERE HE/SHE TEACHES ....

THIS INSTRUCTOR INCORPORATES THE FOLLOWING INTO HIS/HER CLASSES:

☐ INSPIRATIONAL COMMENTARY ☐ HANDS-ON MODIFICATIONS ☐ CHANTING ☐ BREATHING EXERCISES

☐ OTHER: ....

PACE OF FLOW (CIRCLE ONE): FAST MODERATE SLOW

INSTRUCTOR RATINGS: POSE SEQUENCING: CLARITY OF INSTRUCTION: OVERALL RANKING:
A+ A A- B C D F A+ A A- B C D F A+ A A- B C D F

NOTES ....

....

Instructor's name ....

STUDIO/S WHERE HE/SHE TEACHES ....

THIS INSTRUCTOR INCORPORATES THE FOLLOWING INTO HIS/HER CLASSES:

☐ INSPIRATIONAL COMMENTARY ☐ HANDS-ON MODIFICATIONS ☐ CHANTING ☐ BREATHING EXERCISES

☐ OTHER: ....

PACE OF FLOW (CIRCLE ONE): FAST MODERATE SLOW

INSTRUCTOR RATINGS: POSE SEQUENCING: CLARITY OF INSTRUCTION: OVERALL RANKING:
A+ A A- B C D F A+ A A- B C D F A+ A A- B C D F

NOTES ....

....

Instructor's name ....

STUDIO/S WHERE HE/SHE TEACHES ....

THIS INSTRUCTOR INCORPORATES THE FOLLOWING INTO HIS/HER CLASSES:

☐ INSPIRATIONAL COMMENTARY ☐ HANDS-ON MODIFICATIONS ☐ CHANTING ☐ BREATHING EXERCISES

☐ OTHER: ....

PACE OF FLOW (CIRCLE ONE): FAST MODERATE SLOW

INSTRUCTOR RATINGS: POSE SEQUENCING: CLARITY OF INSTRUCTION: OVERALL RANKING:
A+ A A- B C D F A+ A A- B C D F A+ A A- B C D F

NOTES ....

....

One-Year Practice Log

Over the coming twelve-month period, circle the corresponding date every time you practice yoga to create a visual record of how often you practice.

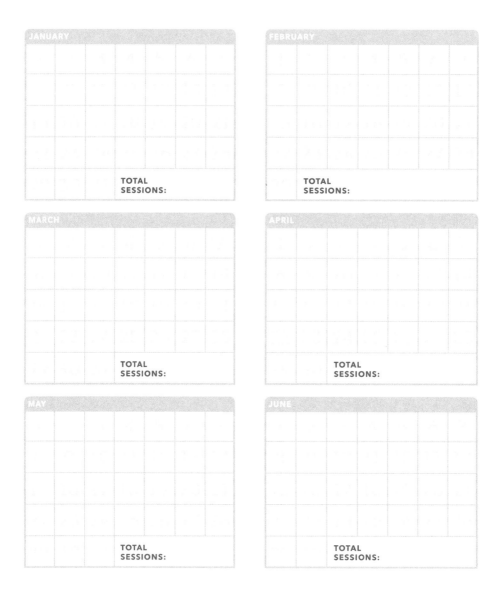

JANUARY

TOTAL SESSIONS:

FEBRUARY

TOTAL SESSIONS:

MARCH

TOTAL SESSIONS:

APRIL

TOTAL SESSIONS:

MAY

TOTAL SESSIONS:

JUNE

TOTAL SESSIONS:

JULY

1	2	3	4	5	6	7
8	9	10	11	12	13	14
15	16	17	18	19	20	21
22	23	24	25	26	27	28
29	30	31				

TOTAL SESSIONS:

AUGUST

1	2	3	4	5	6	7
8	9	10	11	12	13	14
15	16	17	18	19	20	21
22	23	24	25			
29	30	31				

TOTAL SESSIONS:

SEPTEMBER

1	2	3	4	5	6	7
8	9	10	11	12	13	14
15	16	17	18	19	20	21
22	23	24	25	26	27	28
29	30					

TOTAL SESSIONS:

OCTOBER

1	2	3	4	5	6	7
8	9	10	11	12	13	14
15	16	17	18	19	20	21
22	23	24	25	26	27	28
29	30	31				

TOTAL SESSIONS:

NOVEMBER

1	2	3	4	5	6	7
8	9	10	11	12	13	14
15	16	17	18	19	20	21
22	23	24	25	26	27	28

TOTAL SESSIONS:

DECEMBER

1	2	3	4	5	6	7
8	9	10	11	12	13	14
15	16	17	18	19	20	21
22	23	24	25	26	27	28

TOTAL SESSIONS:

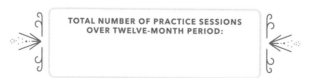

TOTAL NUMBER OF PRACTICE SESSIONS OVER TWELVE-MONTH PERIOD:

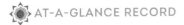

My Dedication Log

Each time you practice yoga, give away your
efforts by dedicating the session to someone
or something that you value in that moment.
Record your dedications here.

DATE OF YOGA SESSION

/   /
....

DEDICATION

....

DATE OF YOGA SESSION

/   /
....

DEDICATION

....

DATE OF YOGA SESSION

/   /
....

DEDICATION

....

DATE OF YOGA SESSION

/   /
....

DEDICATION

....

DATE OF YOGA SESSION

/   /
....

DEDICATION

....

DATE OF YOGA SESSION

/   /
....

DEDICATION

....

DATE OF YOGA SESSION

/   /
....

DEDICATION

....

DATE OF YOGA SESSION

/   /
....

DEDICATION

....

DATE OF YOGA SESSION

/   /
....

DEDICATION

....

DATE OF YOGA SESSION

.... / .... / ....

DEDICATION

....

DATE OF YOGA SESSION

.... / .... / ....

DEDICATION

....

DATE OF YOGA SESSION

.... / .... / ....

DEDICATION

....

DATE OF YOGA SESSION

.... / .... / ....

DEDICATION

....

DATE OF YOGA SESSION

.... / .... / ....

DEDICATION

....

DATE OF YOGA SESSION

.... / .... / ....

DEDICATION

....

DATE OF YOGA SESSION

.... / .... / ....

DEDICATION

....

DATE OF YOGA SESSION

.... / .... / ....

DEDICATION

....

DATE OF YOGA SESSION

.... / .... / ....

DEDICATION

....

DATE OF YOGA SESSION

.... / .... / ....

DEDICATION

....

DATE OF YOGA SESSION

.... / .... / ....

DEDICATION

....

My Yoga Soundtrack

List your favorite pieces of musical accompaniment to create a customized yoga practice soundtrack.

TRACK NAME	ARTIST

TRACK NAME	ARTIST

TRACK NAME	ARTIST

TRACK NAME	ARTIST

TRACK NAME	ARTIST

TRACK NAME	ARTIST

TRACK NAME	ARTIST

TRACK NAME	ARTIST

TRACK NAME	ARTIST

TRACK NAME	ARTIST

TRACK NAME	ARTIST

TRACK NAME	ARTIST

TRACK NAME	ARTIST

TRACK NAME	ARTIST
TRACK NAME	ARTIST
TRACK NAME	ARTIST
TRACK NAME	ARTIST
TRACK NAME	ARTIST
TRACK NAME	ARTIST
TRACK NAME	ARTIST
TRACK NAME	ARTIST
TRACK NAME	ARTIST
TRACK NAME	ARTIST
TRACK NAME	ARTIST
TRACK NAME	ARTIST
TRACK NAME	ARTIST
TRACK NAME	ARTIST
TRACK NAME	ARTIST
TRACK NAME	ARTIST

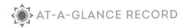

My Collection of Yoga Wisdom

Take note of the wisdom imparted by those in your yoga community—the quotes, affirmations, and positive messages that guide our collective practice to a more meaningful place.

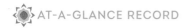
Yoga Around the World

Pinpoint the cities and countries in which you've done yoga and add new marks as you travel for work or play throughout the year. Note the details of these yoga sessions in the pages that follow.

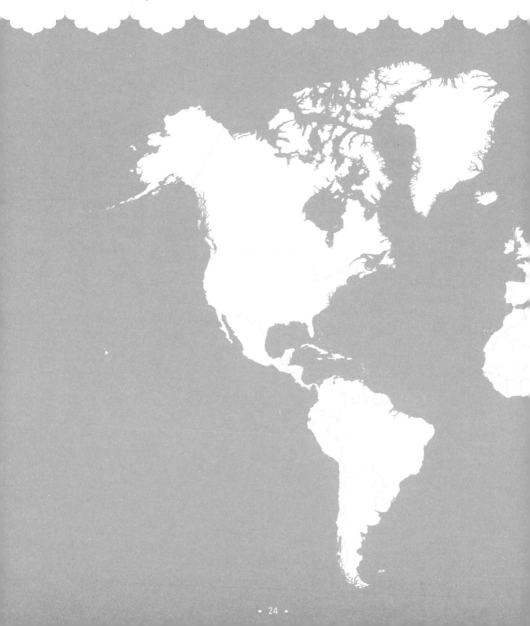

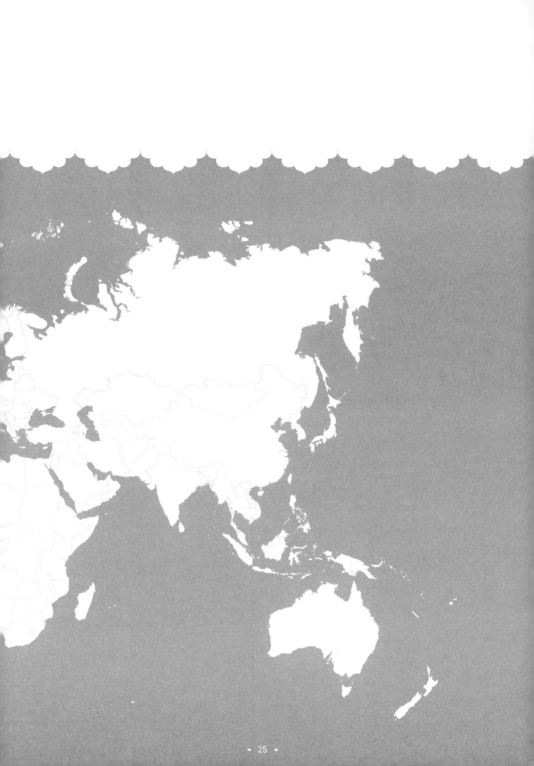

Record the details of your globe-trotting yoga practice,
noting where and when you practiced around the world.

CITY/COUNTRY

MONTH/YEAR

☐ SOLO PRACTICE   ☐ GROUP CLASS

IF GROUP CLASS,
NAME OF STUDIO

NOTES

CITY/COUNTRY

MONTH/YEAR

☐ SOLO PRACTICE   ☐ GROUP CLASS

IF GROUP CLASS,
NAME OF STUDIO

NOTES

CITY/COUNTRY

MONTH/YEAR

☐ SOLO PRACTICE   ☐ GROUP CLASS

IF GROUP CLASS,
NAME OF STUDIO

NOTES

CITY/COUNTRY

MONTH/YEAR

☐ SOLO PRACTICE   ☐ GROUP CLASS

IF GROUP CLASS,
NAME OF STUDIO

NOTES

CITY/COUNTRY

MONTH/YEAR

☐ SOLO PRACTICE ☐ GROUP CLASS

**IF GROUP CLASS,
NAME OF STUDIO**

NOTES

CITY/COUNTRY

MONTH/YEAR

☐ SOLO PRACTICE ☐ GROUP CLASS

**IF GROUP CLASS,
NAME OF STUDIO**

NOTES

CITY/COUNTRY

MONTH/YEAR

☐ SOLO PRACTICE ☐ GROUP CLASS

**IF GROUP CLASS,
NAME OF STUDIO**

NOTES

CITY/COUNTRY

MONTH/YEAR

☐ SOLO PRACTICE ☐ GROUP CLASS

**IF GROUP CLASS,
NAME OF STUDIO**

NOTES

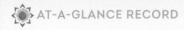
Yoga Gear to Get

ITEM .... HOW THIS MIGHT BENEFIT MY PRACTICE ....

WHERE TO BUY ....

ITEM .... HOW THIS MIGHT BENEFIT MY PRACTICE ....

WHERE TO BUY ....

ITEM .... HOW THIS MIGHT BENEFIT MY PRACTICE ....

WHERE TO BUY ....

ITEM .... HOW THIS MIGHT BENEFIT MY PRACTICE ....

WHERE TO BUY ....

ITEM .... HOW THIS MIGHT BENEFIT MY PRACTICE ....

WHERE TO BUY ....

ITEM .... HOW THIS MIGHT BENEFIT MY PRACTICE ....

WHERE TO BUY ....

ITEM .... HOW THIS MIGHT BENEFIT MY PRACTICE ....

WHERE TO BUY ....

ITEM .... HOW THIS MIGHT BENEFIT MY PRACTICE ....

WHERE TO BUY ....

Yoga Festivals and Events to Check Out

NAME OF EVENT

WHERE

WHEN

HOW THIS MIGHT BENEFIT MY PRACTICE

NAME OF EVENT

WHERE

WHEN

HOW THIS MIGHT BENEFIT MY PRACTICE

NAME OF EVENT

WHERE

WHEN

HOW THIS MIGHT BENEFIT MY PRACTICE

NAME OF EVENT

WHERE

WHEN

HOW THIS MIGHT BENEFIT MY PRACTICE

NAME OF EVENT

WHERE

WHEN

HOW THIS MIGHT BENEFIT MY PRACTICE

NAME OF EVENT

WHERE

WHEN

HOW THIS MIGHT BENEFIT MY PRACTICE

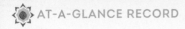

Yoga Books to Read

TITLE ....

AUTHOR ....

HOW THIS MIGHT BENEFIT MY PRACTICE ....
....
....

TITLE ....

AUTHOR ....

HOW THIS MIGHT BENEFIT MY PRACTICE ....
....
....

TITLE ....

AUTHOR ....

HOW THIS MIGHT BENEFIT MY PRACTICE ....
....
....

TITLE ....

AUTHOR ....

HOW THIS MIGHT BENEFIT MY PRACTICE ....
....
....

TITLE ....

AUTHOR ....

HOW THIS MIGHT BENEFIT MY PRACTICE ....
....
....

TITLE ....

AUTHOR ....

HOW THIS MIGHT BENEFIT MY PRACTICE ....
....
....

TITLE ....

AUTHOR ....

HOW THIS MIGHT BENEFIT MY PRACTICE ....
....
....

TITLE ....

AUTHOR ....

HOW THIS MIGHT BENEFIT MY PRACTICE ....
....
....

TITLE ....

AUTHOR ....

HOW THIS MIGHT BENEFIT MY PRACTICE ....
....
....

TITLE ....

AUTHOR ....

HOW THIS MIGHT BENEFIT MY PRACTICE ....
....
....

Yoga Websites to Visit

URL ....

DESCRIPTION ....

HOW THIS MIGHT BENEFIT MY PRACTICE ....
....
....

URL ....

DESCRIPTION ....

HOW THIS MIGHT BENEFIT MY PRACTICE ....
....
....

URL ....

DESCRIPTION ....

HOW THIS MIGHT BENEFIT MY PRACTICE ....
....
....

URL ....

DESCRIPTION ....

HOW THIS MIGHT BENEFIT MY PRACTICE ....
....
....

URL ....

DESCRIPTION ....

HOW THIS MIGHT BENEFIT MY PRACTICE ....
....
....

URL ....

DESCRIPTION ....

HOW THIS MIGHT BENEFIT MY PRACTICE ....
....
....

URL ....

DESCRIPTION ....

HOW THIS MIGHT BENEFIT MY PRACTICE ....
....
....

URL ....

DESCRIPTION ....

HOW THIS MIGHT BENEFIT MY PRACTICE ....
....
....

URL ....

DESCRIPTION ....

HOW THIS MIGHT BENEFIT MY PRACTICE ....
....
....

URL ....

DESCRIPTION ....

HOW THIS MIGHT BENEFIT MY PRACTICE ....
....
....

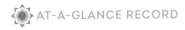 General Health Tracker: Symptoms

Track your physical symptoms. Finding patterns and triggers will help you prevent and manage injuries and improve your yoga experience.

SYMPTOM	FIRST EXPERIENCED	RECURRENCE(S)

POSSIBLE CAUSES	ACTION TAKEN	RESULTS	RESOLVED OR ONGOING?

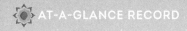
✚ General Health Tracker: Treatments

Record details of visits to health care providers and keep
their contact information handy for future needs.

REASON FOR VISIT

DIAGNOSIS

PRESCRIBED TREATMENT

HEALTH CARE PROVIDER:

NAME ....

SPECIALTY ....

OFFICE ADDRESS ....

....

PHONE ....

DATE

FOLLOW-UP VISIT?   YES   NO

DATE

TAKEAWAYS

COMMENTS

REASON FOR VISIT

DIAGNOSIS

PRESCRIBED TREATMENT

HEALTH CARE PROVIDER:

NAME ....

SPECIALTY ....

OFFICE ADDRESS ....

....

PHONE ....

DATE

FOLLOW-UP VISIT?   YES   NO

DATE

TAKEAWAYS

COMMENTS

REASON FOR VISIT

DIAGNOSIS

PRESCRIBED TREATMENT

HEALTH CARE PROVIDER:

NAME ....

SPECIALTY ....

OFFICE ADDRESS ....

....

PHONE ....

DATE

FOLLOW-UP VISIT?   YES   NO

DATE

TAKEAWAYS

COMMENTS

REASON FOR VISIT

DIAGNOSIS

PRESCRIBED TREATMENT

HEALTH CARE PROVIDER:

NAME ....

SPECIALTY ....

OFFICE ADDRESS ....

....

PHONE ....

DATE

FOLLOW-UP VISIT?   YES   NO

DATE

TAKEAWAYS

COMMENTS

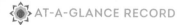

General Health Tracker:
Medications and Nutritional Supplements

Monitor your medications and nutritional supplements to track your health and healing, and to understand your patterns of use.

MEDICATION/SUPPLEMENT

DATE STARTED

USED FOR

DOSAGE

EFFECT

MEDICATION/SUPPLEMENT

DATE STARTED

USED FOR

DOSAGE

EFFECT

MEDICATION/SUPPLEMENT

DATE STARTED

USED FOR

DOSAGE

EFFECT

MEDICATION/SUPPLEMENT

DATE STARTED

USED FOR

DOSAGE

EFFECT

MEDICATION/SUPPLEMENT

DATE STARTED

USED FOR

DOSAGE

EFFECT

MEDICATION/SUPPLEMENT

DATE STARTED

USED FOR

DOSAGE

EFFECT

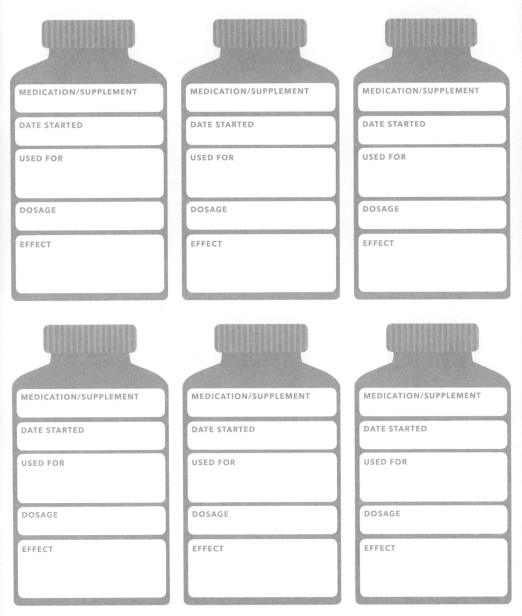

MEDICATION/SUPPLEMENT

DATE STARTED

USED FOR

DOSAGE

EFFECT

MEDICATION/SUPPLEMENT

DATE STARTED

USED FOR

DOSAGE

EFFECT

MEDICATION/SUPPLEMENT

DATE STARTED

USED FOR

DOSAGE

EFFECT

MEDICATION/SUPPLEMENT

DATE STARTED

USED FOR

DOSAGE

EFFECT

MEDICATION/SUPPLEMENT

DATE STARTED

USED FOR

DOSAGE

EFFECT

MEDICATION/SUPPLEMENT

DATE STARTED

USED FOR

DOSAGE

EFFECT

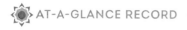 For Yoga Moms: My Prenatal Practice

As a supplement to other prenatal care, prenatal yoga can help support your body's changing needs and prepare you for the birth of your baby. Track your practice, and key aspects of your pregnancy, here.

DUE DATE / /

Important Contacts

CARE PROVIDER

OTHER SUPPORT PROVIDER

CONTACT INFO

CONTACT INFO

☐ DOCTOR ☐ MIDWIFE ☐ DOULA ☐ OTHER ....

☐ DOCTOR ☐ MIDWIFE ☐ DOULA ☐ OTHER ....

HAVE ANY EXERCISE-RELATED RESTRICTIONS OR PRECAUTIONS BEEN ADVISED BY YOUR CARE PROVIDERS?

☐ YES ☐ NO   **IF YES, LIST THEM HERE** ....

Pregnancy Symptoms

CHECK OFF THE SYMPTOMS YOU'VE HAD IN YOUR FIRST, SECOND, AND THIRD TRIMESTER AND ASK YOUR INSTRUCTOR FOR SPECIFIC POSES THAT ARE RECOMMENDED FOR SYMPTOM RELIEF.

	1ST	2ND	3RD	RECOMMENDED POSE
NAUSEA				
FATIGUE				
INDIGESTION				
ANXIETY				
INSOMNIA				
BACKACHES				
HEADACHES				
OTHER				
OTHER				

FAVORITE PRENATAL YOGA POSES

1. ....

2. ....

3. ....

POSES YOU MIGHT USE DURING CHILDBIRTH

1. ....

2. ....

3. ....

Prenatal Practice Log

RECORD THE DETAILS OF EACH PRENATAL YOGA SESSION.

DATE   /   /   TIME   -

LOCATION

INSTRUCTOR

NOTES

DATE   /   /   TIME   -

LOCATION

INSTRUCTOR

NOTES

DATE   /   /   TIME   -

LOCATION

INSTRUCTOR

NOTES

DATE   /   /   TIME   -

LOCATION

INSTRUCTOR

NOTES

DATE   /   /   TIME   -

LOCATION

INSTRUCTOR

NOTES

DATE   /   /   TIME   -

LOCATION

INSTRUCTOR

NOTES

DATE   /   /   TIME   -

LOCATION

INSTRUCTOR

NOTES

DATE   /   /   TIME   -

LOCATION

INSTRUCTOR

NOTES

DATE   /   /   TIME   -

LOCATION

INSTRUCTOR

NOTES

DATE   /   /   TIME   -

LOCATION

INSTRUCTOR

NOTES

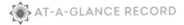 For Yoga Moms: My Postnatal Practice

Return to this section after the birth of your baby and track your postnatal practice. *Note: Medical professionals recommend waiting at least six weeks before attempting any form of physical exercise. Consult your health care provider before resuming or starting a yoga practice.*

NAME OF YOUR BABY

BIRTH DATE

Postnatal Practice Log

DATE   /   /   **TIME**   -

LOCATION

INSTRUCTOR

NOTES

DATE   /   /   **TIME**   -

LOCATION

INSTRUCTOR

NOTES

DATE   /   /   **TIME**   -

LOCATION

INSTRUCTOR

NOTES

DATE   /   /   **TIME**   -

LOCATION

INSTRUCTOR

NOTES

DATE   /   /   **TIME**   -

LOCATION

INSTRUCTOR

NOTES

DATE   /   /   **TIME**   -

LOCATION

INSTRUCTOR

NOTES

DATE   /   /   TIME   -

LOCATION

INSTRUCTOR

NOTES

DATE   /   /   TIME   -

LOCATION

INSTRUCTOR

NOTES

DATE   /   /   TIME   -

LOCATION

INSTRUCTOR

NOTES

DATE   /   /   TIME   -

LOCATION

INSTRUCTOR

NOTES

DATE   /   /   TIME   -

LOCATION

INSTRUCTOR

NOTES

DATE   /   /   TIME   -

LOCATION

INSTRUCTOR

NOTES

DATE   /   /   TIME   -

LOCATION

INSTRUCTOR

NOTES

DATE   /   /   TIME   -

LOCATION

INSTRUCTOR

NOTES

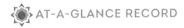

My Goals

List your goals (short-term and long-term, yoga-related or not) for an inspirational record of the ways you aim to reach your potential, on and off the mat.

1. _____

2. _____

3. _____

4. _____

5. _____

6. _____

7. _____

8. _____

9. _____

10. _____

11. _____

12. _____

Yoga Session Journal

Record the details of
forty-five individual yoga
sessions in the pages ahead
and witness the deepening
of your practice.

Yoga Session ①

DATE   /   /   TIME   -

☐ **Group Class Practice**   ☐ **Home Practice and/or**
                                                  Private Instruction

NAME OF STUDIO: (OR)   IN WHAT ROOM/SPACE DID YOU PRACTICE?

NAME OF TEACHER:

TEACHER RATING (CIRCLE ONE): A+ A A- B C D F   ON WHAT PART OF THE BODY DID YOU FOCUS
                                                        DURING THIS SESSION?
CLASS LEVEL:
☐ BEGINNER   ☐ INTERMEDIATE   ☐ ADVANCED   ☐ ABDOMINALS   ☐ HIPS
                                                     ☐ BACK   ☐ BUTTOCKS
CROWD LEVEL: 1 2 3 4 5   ☐ SHOULDERS   ☐ LEGS
           NOT CROWDED > CROWDED   ☐ ARMS   ☐ ANKLES/FEET
TEMPERATURE: ☐ HEATED   ☐ UNHEATED   ☐ WRISTS/HANDS ☐ OTHER:

Session Details

WHAT STYLE DID YOU PRACTICE DURING THIS SESSION?   WHAT TOOLS DID YOU HAVE ON HAND?
☐ ANUSARA   ☐ KRIPALU   ☐ MAT   ☐ STRAP
☐ ASHTANGA   ☐ KUNDALINI   ☐ WATER BOTTLE ☐ BLANKET
☐ BIKRAM   ☐ POWER   ☐ TOWEL   ☐ BOLSTER PILLOW
☐ IYENGAR   ☐ RESTORATIVE   ☐ BLOCK   ☐ OTHER:
☐ JIVAMUKTI   ☐ VINIYOGA
                 ☐ OTHER:

SOUND ACCOMPANIMENT: ☐ NO MUSIC   ☐ MUSIC

FAVORITE TRACK FROM TODAY'S SESSION
[DOWNLOAD THIS ONE AND THE SONGS TO YOUR YOGA SOUND TRACK!]

Overall Session Rating

PACE OF FLOW: 1 2 3 4 5   FAVORITE POSE OF TODAY'S SESSION:

DYNAMISM OF   1 2 3 4 5
SEQUENCING: MOST CHALLENGING POSE:

DIFFICULTY: 1 2 3 4 5
                                         POSE YOU HADN'T TRIED BEFORE TODAY:
POSES INCLUDED IN TODAY'S SEQUENCING:

☐ STANDING POSES   ☐ FORWARD BENDS
☐ BALANCING POSES   ☐ BACKBENDS   POSE IN WHICH YOU SHOWED THE MOST IMPROVEMENT:
☐ SEATED POSES   ☐ INVERSIONS
☐ ABDOMINAL   ☐ RESTING POSES
  STRENGTHENERS   POSE YOU'D LIKE TO WORK ON IN THE NEXT SESSION:
☐ TWISTS

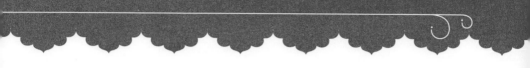

Dedication

TO WHOM OR WHAT DID YOU DEDICATE THIS CLASS?
(TURN TO PAGE 18 AND ADD YOUR ANSWER TO YOUR DEDICATION LOG.)

Notes and Takeaways

Self-Review

One a scale of 1 to 5 (low to high), rate the following areas of your performance during this session:

FOCUS: 1 2 3 4 5

EVENNESS
OF BREATH: 1 2 3 4 5

BALANCE: 1 2 3 4 5

STRENGTH: 1 2 3 4 5

ENERGY
LEVEL: 1 2 3 4 5

ATTITUDE: 1 2 3 4 5

Yoga Session 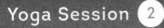 2

DATE   /   /   **TIME**   -

☐ **Group Class Practice**

☐ **Home Practice and/or Private Instruction**

NAME OF STUDIO:

(OR)   **IN WHAT ROOM/SPACE DID YOU PRACTICE?**

NAME OF TEACHER:

TEACHER RATING (CIRCLE ONE): A+ A A- B C D F

ON WHAT PART OF THE BODY DID YOU FOCUS DURING THIS SESSION?

CLASS LEVEL:
☐ BEGINNER   ☐ INTERMEDIATE   ☐ ADVANCED

CROWD LEVEL: ① ② ③ ④ ⑤
    NOT CROWDED ▸ CROWDED

TEMPERATURE: ☐ HEATED   ☐ UNHEATED

☐ ABDOMINALS   ☐ HIPS
☐ BACK   ☐ BUTTOCKS
☐ SHOULDERS   ☐ LEGS
☐ ARMS   ☐ ANKLES/FEET
☐ WRISTS/HANDS ☐ OTHER:

Session Details

WHAT STYLE DID YOU PRACTICE DURING THIS SESSION?

☐ ANUSARA   ☐ KRIPALU
☐ ASHTANGA   ☐ KUNDALINI
☐ BIKRAM   ☐ POWER
☐ IYENGAR   ☐ RESTORATIVE
☐ JIVAMUKTI   ☐ VINIYOGA
                ☐ OTHER:

WHAT TOOLS DID YOU HAVE ON HAND?

☐ MAT   ☐ STRAP
☐ WATER BOTTLE   ☐ BLANKET
☐ TOWEL   ☐ BOLSTER PILLOW
☐ BLOCK   ☐ OTHER:

SOUND ACCOMPANIMENT: ☐ NO MUSIC   ☐ MUSIC

FAVORITE TRACK FROM TODAY'S SESSION
(TURN TO PAGE 20 AND ADD THE SONG TO YOUR YOGA SOUNDTRACK.)

Overall Session Rating

PACE OF FLOW: ① ② ③ ④ ⑤

FAVORITE POSE OF TODAY'S SESSION:

DYNAMISM OF SEQUENCING: ① ② ③ ④ ⑤

MOST CHALLENGING POSE:

DIFFICULTY: ① ② ③ ④ ⑤

POSES INCLUDED IN TODAY'S SEQUENCING:

☐ STANDING POSES   ☐ FORWARD BENDS
☐ BALANCING POSES   ☐ BACKBENDS
☐ SEATED POSES   ☐ INVERSIONS
☐ ABDOMINAL   ☐ RESTING POSES
   STRENGTHENERS
☐ TWISTS

POSE YOU HADN'T TRIED BEFORE TODAY:

POSE IN WHICH YOU SHOWED THE MOST IMPROVEMENT:

POSE YOU'D LIKE TO WORK ON IN THE NEXT SESSION:

Dedication

TO WHOM OR WHAT DID YOU DEDICATE THIS CLASS?
(TURN TO PAGE 18 AND ADD YOUR ANSWER TO YOUR DEDICATION LOG.)

Notes and Takeaways

Self-Review

One a scale of 1 to 5 (low to high), rate the following areas of your performance during this session:

FOCUS: 1 2 3 4 5

EVENNESS OF BREATH: 1 2 3 4 5

BALANCE: 1 2 3 4 5

STRENGTH: 1 2 3 4 5

ENERGY LEVEL: 1 2 3 4 5

ATTITUDE: 1 2 3 4 5

DATE / / **TIME** -

☐ **Group Class Practice**

☐ **Home Practice and/or Private Instruction**

NAME OF STUDIO:

(OR)   IN WHAT ROOM/SPACE DID YOU PRACTICE?

NAME OF TEACHER:

TEACHER RATING (CIRCLE ONE): A+ A A- B C D F

CLASS LEVEL:
☐ BEGINNER ☐ INTERMEDIATE ☐ ADVANCED

CROWD LEVEL: 1 2 3 4 5
        NOT CROWDED ▸ CROWDED

TEMPERATURE: ☐ HEATED ☐ UNHEATED

ON WHAT PART OF THE BODY DID YOU FOCUS DURING THIS SESSION?
☐ ABDOMINALS ☐ HIPS
☐ BACK ☐ BUTTOCKS
☐ SHOULDERS ☐ LEGS
☐ ARMS ☐ ANKLES/FEET
☐ WRISTS/HANDS ☐ OTHER:

Session Details

WHAT STYLE DID YOU PRACTICE DURING THIS SESSION?
☐ ANUSARA ☐ KRIPALU
☐ ASHTANGA ☐ KUNDALINI
☐ BIKRAM ☐ POWER
☐ IYENGAR ☐ RESTORATIVE
☐ JIVAMUKTI ☐ VINIYOGA
        ☐ OTHER:

WHAT TOOLS DID YOU HAVE ON HAND?
☐ MAT ☐ STRAP
☐ WATER BOTTLE ☐ BLANKET
☐ TOWEL ☐ BOLSTER PILLOW
☐ BLOCK ☐ OTHER:

SOUND ACCOMPANIMENT: ☐ NO MUSIC ☐ MUSIC

FAVORITE TRACK FROM TODAY'S SESSION
(TURN TO PAGE 20 AND ADD THE SONG TO YOUR YOGA SOUNDTRACK.)

Overall Session Rating

PACE OF FLOW: 1 2 3 4 5

DYNAMISM OF SEQUENCING: 1 2 3 4 5

DIFFICULTY: 1 2 3 4 5

POSES INCLUDED IN TODAY'S SEQUENCING:
☐ STANDING POSES ☐ FORWARD BENDS
☐ BALANCING POSES ☐ BACKBENDS
☐ SEATED POSES ☐ INVERSIONS
☐ ABDOMINAL STRENGTHENERS ☐ RESTING POSES
☐ TWISTS

FAVORITE POSE OF TODAY'S SESSION:

MOST CHALLENGING POSE:

POSE YOU HADN'T TRIED BEFORE TODAY:

POSE IN WHICH YOU SHOWED THE MOST IMPROVEMENT:

POSE YOU'D LIKE TO WORK ON IN THE NEXT SESSION:

Dedication

TO WHOM OR WHAT DID YOU DEDICATE THIS CLASS?

(TURN TO PAGE 18 AND ADD YOUR ANSWER TO YOUR DEDICATION LOG.)

Notes and Takeaways

Self-Review

One a scale of 1 to 5 (low to high), rate the following areas of your performance during this session:

FOCUS: 1 2 3 4 5

EVENNESS
OF BREATH: 1 2 3 4 5

BALANCE: 1 2 3 4 5

STRENGTH: 1 2 3 4 5

ENERGY
LEVEL: 1 2 3 4 5

ATTITUDE: 1 2 3 4 5

DATE   /   /   **TIME**   -

☐ **Group Class Practice**   ☐ **Home Practice and/or
                                                  Private Instruction**

NAME OF STUDIO: _____   (OR)   IN WHAT ROOM/SPACE DID YOU PRACTICE?

NAME OF TEACHER: _____

TEACHER RATING (CIRCLE ONE): A+ A A- B C D F   ON WHAT PART OF THE BODY DID YOU FOCUS
                                                 DURING THIS SESSION?
CLASS LEVEL:
☐ BEGINNER ☐ INTERMEDIATE ☐ ADVANCED   ☐ ABDOMINALS   ☐ HIPS
                                                 ☐ BACK   ☐ BUTTOCKS
CROWD LEVEL: 1 2 3 4 5   ☐ SHOULDERS   ☐ LEGS
              NOT CROWDED → CROWDED   ☐ ARMS   ☐ ANKLES/FEET
TEMPERATURE: ☐ HEATED ☐ UNHEATED   ☐ WRISTS/HANDS   ☐ OTHER:

Session Details

WHAT STYLE DID YOU PRACTICE DURING THIS SESSION?   WHAT TOOLS DID YOU HAVE ON HAND?
☐ ANUSARA   ☐ KRIPALU   ☐ MAT   ☐ STRAP
☐ ASHTANGA   ☐ KUNDALINI   ☐ WATER BOTTLE   ☐ BLANKET
☐ BIKRAM   ☐ POWER   ☐ TOWEL   ☐ BOLSTER PILLOW
☐ IYENGAR   ☐ RESTORATIVE   ☐ BLOCK   ☐ OTHER:
☐ JIVAMUKTI   ☐ VINIYOGA
                 ☐ OTHER:

SOUND ACCOMPANIMENT: ☐ NO MUSIC   ☐ MUSIC

FAVORITE TRACK FROM TODAY'S SESSION
(TURN TO PAGE 20 AND ADD THE SONG TO YOUR YOGA SOUNDTRACK)

Overall Session Rating

PACE OF FLOW: 1 2 3 4 5   FAVORITE POSE OF TODAY'S SESSION:

DYNAMISM OF   1 2 3 4 5
SEQUENCING:
                                       MOST CHALLENGING POSE:
DIFFICULTY: 1 2 3 4 5

POSES INCLUDED IN TODAY'S SEQUENCING: POSE YOU HADN'T TRIED BEFORE TODAY:

☐ STANDING POSES   ☐ FORWARD BENDS
☐ BALANCING POSES   ☐ BACKBENDS
☐ SEATED POSES   ☐ INVERSIONS   POSE IN WHICH YOU SHOWED THE MOST IMPROVEMENT:
☐ ABDOMINAL   ☐ RESTING POSES
  STRENGTHENERS
☐ TWISTS   POSE YOU'D LIKE TO WORK ON IN THE NEXT SESSION:

Dedication

TO WHOM OR WHAT DID YOU DEDICATE THIS CLASS?
(TURN TO PAGE 18 AND ADD YOUR ANSWER TO YOUR DEDICATION LOG.)

Notes and Takeaways

Self-Review

One a scale of 1 to 5 (low to high), rate the following areas of your performance during this session:

FOCUS: 1 2 3 4 5

EVENNESS
OF BREATH: 1 2 3 4 5

BALANCE: 1 2 3 4 5

STRENGTH: 1 2 3 4 5

ENERGY
LEVEL: 1 2 3 4 5

ATTITUDE: 1 2 3 4 5

DATE   /   /   TIME   -

☐ **Group Class Practice**   ☐ **Home Practice and/or**
                                                    Private Instruction

NAME OF STUDIO: _____   (OR)   IN WHAT ROOM/SPACE DID YOU PRACTICE?

NAME OF TEACHER: _____

TEACHER RATING (CIRCLE ONE): A+ A A- B C D F   ON WHAT PART OF THE BODY DID YOU FOCUS
                                                        DURING THIS SESSION?
CLASS LEVEL:
☐ BEGINNER   ☐ INTERMEDIATE   ☐ ADVANCED   ☐ ABDOMINALS   ☐ HIPS
                                                    ☐ BACK   ☐ BUTTOCKS
CROWD LEVEL: ①②③④⑤   ☐ SHOULDERS   ☐ LEGS
           NOT CROWDED ▶ CROWDED   ☐ ARMS   ☐ ANKLES/FEET

TEMPERATURE: ☐ HEATED   ☐ UNHEATED   ☐ WRISTS/HANDS   ☐ OTHER: _____

Session Details

WHAT STYLE DID YOU PRACTICE DURING THIS SESSION?   WHAT TOOLS DID YOU HAVE ON HAND?
☐ ANUSARA   ☐ KRIPALU   ☐ MAT   ☐ STRAP
☐ ASHTANGA   ☐ KUNDALINI   ☐ WATER BOTTLE   ☐ BLANKET
☐ BIKRAM   ☐ POWER   ☐ TOWEL   ☐ BOLSTER PILLOW
☐ IYENGAR   ☐ RESTORATIVE   ☐ BLOCK   ☐ OTHER: _____
☐ JIVAMUKTI   ☐ VINIYOGA
                  ☐ OTHER: _____

SOUND ACCOMPANIMENT: ☐ NO MUSIC   ☐ MUSIC

FAVORITE TRACK FROM TODAY'S SESSION _____
(TURN TO PAGE 20 AND ADD THE SONG TO YOUR YOGA SOUNDTRACK.)

Overall Session Rating

PACE OF FLOW: ①②③④⑤   FAVORITE POSE OF TODAY'S SESSION:

DYNAMISM OF   ①②③④⑤
SEQUENCING: MOST CHALLENGING POSE:

DIFFICULTY: ①②③④⑤

POSES INCLUDED IN TODAY'S SEQUENCING: POSE YOU HADN'T TRIED BEFORE TODAY:

☐ STANDING POSES   ☐ FORWARD BENDS
☐ BALANCING POSES   ☐ BACKBENDS   POSE IN WHICH YOU SHOWED THE MOST IMPROVEMENT:
☐ SEATED POSES   ☐ INVERSIONS
☐ ABDOMINAL   ☐ RESTING POSES
   STRENGTHENERS   POSE YOU'D LIKE TO WORK ON IN THE NEXT SESSION:
☐ TWISTS

Dedication

TO WHOM OR WHAT DID YOU DEDICATE THIS CLASS?
(TURN TO PAGE 18 AND ADD YOUR ANSWER TO YOUR DEDICATION LOG.)

Notes and Takeaways

Self-Review

One a scale of 1 to 5 (low to high), rate the following areas of your performance during this session:

FOCUS: 1 2 3 4 5

EVENNESS OF BREATH: 1 2 3 4 5

BALANCE: 1 2 3 4 5

STRENGTH: 1 2 3 4 5

ENERGY LEVEL: 1 2 3 4 5

ATTITUDE: 1 2 3 4 5

DATE / /   **TIME** -

☐ **Group Class Practice**

NAME OF STUDIO:

NAME OF TEACHER:

TEACHER RATING (CIRCLE ONE): A+ A A- B C D F

CLASS LEVEL:
☐ BEGINNER ☐ INTERMEDIATE ☐ ADVANCED

CROWD LEVEL: 1 2 3 4 5
           NOT CROWDED ▸ CROWDED

TEMPERATURE: ☐ HEATED ☐ UNHEATED

(OR)

☐ **Home Practice and/or Private Instruction**

IN WHAT ROOM/SPACE DID YOU PRACTICE?

ON WHAT PART OF THE BODY DID YOU FOCUS DURING THIS SESSION?
☐ ABDOMINALS ☐ HIPS
☐ BACK ☐ BUTTOCKS
☐ SHOULDERS ☐ LEGS
☐ ARMS ☐ ANKLES/FEET
☐ WRISTS/HANDS ☐ OTHER:

Session Details

WHAT STYLE DID YOU PRACTICE DURING THIS SESSION?
☐ ANUSARA ☐ KRIPALU
☐ ASHTANGA ☐ KUNDALINI
☐ BIKRAM ☐ POWER
☐ IYENGAR ☐ RESTORATIVE
☐ JIVAMUKTI ☐ VINIYOGA
☐ OTHER:

WHAT TOOLS DID YOU HAVE ON HAND?
☐ MAT ☐ STRAP
☐ WATER BOTTLE ☐ BLANKET
☐ TOWEL ☐ BOLSTER PILLOW
☐ BLOCK ☐ OTHER:

SOUND ACCOMPANIMENT: ☐ NO MUSIC ☐ MUSIC

FAVORITE TRACK FROM TODAY'S SESSION
(TURN TO PAGE 20 AND ADD THE SONG TO YOUR YOGA SOUNDTRACK.)

Overall Session Rating

PACE OF FLOW: 1 2 3 4 5

DYNAMISM OF SEQUENCING: 1 2 3 4 5

DIFFICULTY: 1 2 3 4 5

POSES INCLUDED IN TODAY'S SEQUENCING:
☐ STANDING POSES ☐ FORWARD BENDS
☐ BALANCING POSES ☐ BACKBENDS
☐ SEATED POSES ☐ INVERSIONS
☐ ABDOMINAL STRENGTHENERS ☐ RESTING POSES
☐ TWISTS

FAVORITE POSE OF TODAY'S SESSION:

MOST CHALLENGING POSE:

POSE YOU HADN'T TRIED BEFORE TODAY:

POSE IN WHICH YOU SHOWED THE MOST IMPROVEMENT:

POSE YOU'D LIKE TO WORK ON IN THE NEXT SESSION:

Dedication

TO WHOM OR WHAT DID YOU DEDICATE THIS CLASS?
(TURN TO PAGE 18 AND ADD YOUR ANSWER TO YOUR DEDICATION LOG.)

Notes and Takeaways

Self-Review

One a scale of 1 to 5 (low to high), rate the following areas of your performance during this session:

FOCUS: 1 2 3 4 5

EVENNESS
OF BREATH: 1 2 3 4 5

BALANCE: 1 2 3 4 5

STRENGTH: 1 2 3 4 5

ENERGY
LEVEL: 1 2 3 4 5

ATTITUDE: 1 2 3 4 5

Yoga Session 7

DATE   /   /   TIME   -

☐ **Group Class Practice**

☐ **Home Practice and/or Private Instruction**

(OR)

NAME OF STUDIO: 　　　　　　IN WHAT ROOM/SPACE DID YOU PRACTICE?

NAME OF TEACHER:

TEACHER RATING (CIRCLE ONE): A+ A A- B C D F

CLASS LEVEL:
☐ BEGINNER ☐ INTERMEDIATE ☐ ADVANCED

CROWD LEVEL: (1) (2) (3) (4) (5)
　　　　NOT CROWDED ▸ CROWDED

TEMPERATURE: ☐ HEATED ☐ UNHEATED

ON WHAT PART OF THE BODY DID YOU FOCUS DURING THIS SESSION?
☐ ABDOMINALS ☐ HIPS
☐ BACK ☐ BUTTOCKS
☐ SHOULDERS ☐ LEGS
☐ ARMS ☐ ANKLES/FEET
☐ WRISTS/HANDS ☐ OTHER:

Session Details

WHAT STYLE DID YOU PRACTICE DURING THIS SESSION?
☐ ANUSARA ☐ KRIPALU
☐ ASHTANGA ☐ KUNDALINI
☐ BIKRAM ☐ POWER
☐ IYENGAR ☐ RESTORATIVE
☐ JIVAMUKTI ☐ VINIYOGA
　　　　☐ OTHER:

WHAT TOOLS DID YOU HAVE ON HAND?
☐ MAT ☐ STRAP
☐ WATER BOTTLE ☐ BLANKET
☐ TOWEL ☐ BOLSTER PILLOW
☐ BLOCK ☐ OTHER:

SOUND ACCOMPANIMENT: ☐ NO MUSIC ☐ MUSIC

FAVORITE TRACK FROM TODAY'S SESSION
(TURN TO PAGE 20 AND ADD THE SONG TO YOUR YOGA SOUNDTRACK.)

Overall Session Rating

PACE OF FLOW: (1) (2) (3) (4) (5)

DYNAMISM OF SEQUENCING: (1) (2) (3) (4) (5)

DIFFICULTY: (1) (2) (3) (4) (5)

POSES INCLUDED IN TODAY'S SEQUENCING:
☐ STANDING POSES ☐ FORWARD BENDS
☐ BALANCING POSES ☐ BACKBENDS
☐ SEATED POSES ☐ INVERSIONS
☐ ABDOMINAL STRENGTHENERS ☐ RESTING POSES
☐ TWISTS

FAVORITE POSE OF TODAY'S SESSION:

MOST CHALLENGING POSE:

POSE YOU HADN'T TRIED BEFORE TODAY:

POSE IN WHICH YOU SHOWED THE MOST IMPROVEMENT:

POSE YOU'D LIKE TO WORK ON IN THE NEXT SESSION:

Dedication

TO WHOM OR WHAT DID YOU DEDICATE THIS CLASS?
(TURN TO PAGE 18 AND ADD YOUR ANSWER TO YOUR DEDICATION LOG.)

Notes and Takeaways

Self-Review

One a scale of 1 to 5 (low to high), rate the following areas of your performance during this session:

FOCUS: ① ② ③ ④ ⑤

EVENNESS OF BREATH: ① ② ③ ④ ⑤

BALANCE: ① ② ③ ④ ⑤

STRENGTH: ① ② ③ ④ ⑤

ENERGY LEVEL: ① ② ③ ④ ⑤

ATTITUDE: ① ② ③ ④ ⑤

DATE   /   /   TIME   -

☐ **Group Class Practice**   ☐ **Home Practice and/or Private Instruction**

NAME OF STUDIO: (OR)   IN WHAT ROOM/SPACE DID YOU PRACTICE?

NAME OF TEACHER:

TEACHER RATING (CIRCLE ONE): A+ A A- B C D F   ON WHAT PART OF THE BODY DID YOU FOCUS DURING THIS SESSION?

CLASS LEVEL:
☐ BEGINNER   ☐ INTERMEDIATE   ☐ ADVANCED   ☐ ABDOMINALS   ☐ HIPS
                                                 ☐ BACK   ☐ BUTTOCKS
CROWD LEVEL: 1 2 3 4 5   ☐ SHOULDERS   ☐ LEGS
          NOT CROWDED ► CROWDED   ☐ ARMS   ☐ ANKLES/FEET

TEMPERATURE: ☐ HEATED   ☐ UNHEATED   ☐ WRISTS/HANDS ☐ OTHER:

Session Details

WHAT STYLE DID YOU PRACTICE DURING THIS SESSION?   WHAT TOOLS DID YOU HAVE ON HAND?

☐ ANUSARA   ☐ KRIPALU   ☐ MAT   ☐ STRAP
☐ ASHTANGA   ☐ KUNDALINI   ☐ WATER BOTTLE   ☐ BLANKET
☐ BIKRAM   ☐ POWER   ☐ TOWEL   ☐ BOLSTER PILLOW
☐ IYENGAR   ☐ RESTORATIVE   ☐ BLOCK   ☐ OTHER:
☐ JIVAMUKTI   ☐ VINIYOGA
                 ☐ OTHER:

SOUND ACCOMPANIMENT: ☐ NO MUSIC   ☐ MUSIC -

FAVORITE TRACK FROM TODAY'S SESSION
(TURN TO PAGE 20 AND ADD THE SONG TO YOUR YOGA SOUNDTRACK.)

Overall Session Rating

PACE OF FLOW: 1 2 3 4 5   FAVORITE POSE OF TODAY'S SESSION:

DYNAMISM OF   1 2 3 4 5
SEQUENCING: MOST CHALLENGING POSE:

DIFFICULTY: 1 2 3 4 5

POSES INCLUDED IN TODAY'S SEQUENCING: POSE YOU HADN'T TRIED BEFORE TODAY:

☐ STANDING POSES   ☐ FORWARD BENDS
☐ BALANCING POSES   ☐ BACKBENDS   POSE IN WHICH YOU SHOWED THE MOST IMPROVEMENT:
☐ SEATED POSES   ☐ INVERSIONS
☐ ABDOMINAL   ☐ RESTING POSES
  STRENGTHENERS   POSE YOU'D LIKE TO WORK ON IN THE NEXT SESSION:
☐ TWISTS

Dedication

TO WHOM OR WHAT DID YOU DEDICATE THIS CLASS?
(TURN TO PAGE 18 AND ADD YOUR ANSWER TO YOUR DEDICATION LOG.)

Notes and Takeaways

Self-Review

One a scale of 1 to 5 (low to high), rate the following areas of your performance during this session:

FOCUS: 1 2 3 4 5

EVENNESS
OF BREATH: 1 2 3 4 5

BALANCE: 1 2 3 4 5

STRENGTH: 1 2 3 4 5

ENERGY
LEVEL: 1 2 3 4 5

ATTITUDE: 1 2 3 4 5

Yoga Session ⑨

DATE   /   /   TIME   -

☐ **Group Class Practice**

NAME OF STUDIO:

NAME OF TEACHER:

TEACHER RATING (CIRCLE ONE): A+ A A- B C D F

CLASS LEVEL:
☐ BEGINNER   ☐ INTERMEDIATE   ☐ ADVANCED

CROWD LEVEL: ① ② ③ ④ ⑤
              NOT CROWDED ▶ CROWDED

TEMPERATURE: ☐ HEATED   ☐ UNHEATED

OR

☐ **Home Practice and/or Private Instruction**

IN WHAT ROOM/SPACE DID YOU PRACTICE?

ON WHAT PART OF THE BODY DID YOU FOCUS DURING THIS SESSION?
☐ ABDOMINALS   ☐ HIPS
☐ BACK   ☐ BUTTOCKS
☐ SHOULDERS   ☐ LEGS
☐ ARMS   ☐ ANKLES/FEET
☐ WRISTS/HANDS   ☐ OTHER:

Session Details

WHAT STYLE DID YOU PRACTICE DURING THIS SESSION?
☐ ANUSARA   ☐ KRIPALU
☐ ASHTANGA   ☐ KUNDALINI
☐ BIKRAM   ☐ POWER
☐ IYENGAR   ☐ RESTORATIVE
☐ JIVAMUKTI   ☐ VINIYOGA
                 ☐ OTHER:

WHAT TOOLS DID YOU HAVE ON HAND?
☐ MAT   ☐ STRAP
☐ WATER BOTTLE   ☐ BLANKET
☐ TOWEL   ☐ BOLSTER PILLOW
☐ BLOCK   ☐ OTHER:

SOUND ACCOMPANIMENT: ☐ NO MUSIC   ☐ MUSIC

FAVORITE TRACK FROM TODAY'S SESSION
(TURN TO PAGE 20 AND ADD THE SONG TO YOUR YOGA SOUNDTRACK.)

Overall Session Rating

PACE OF FLOW: ① ② ③ ④ ⑤

DYNAMISM OF SEQUENCING: ① ② ③ ④ ⑤

DIFFICULTY: ① ② ③ ④ ⑤

POSES INCLUDED IN TODAY'S SEQUENCING:
☐ STANDING POSES   ☐ FORWARD BENDS
☐ BALANCING POSES   ☐ BACKBENDS
☐ SEATED POSES   ☐ INVERSIONS
☐ ABDOMINAL STRENGTHENERS   ☐ RESTING POSES
☐ TWISTS

FAVORITE POSE OF TODAY'S SESSION:

MOST CHALLENGING POSE:

POSE YOU HADN'T TRIED BEFORE TODAY:

POSE IN WHICH YOU SHOWED THE MOST IMPROVEMENT:

POSE YOU'D LIKE TO WORK ON IN THE NEXT SESSION:

Dedication

TO WHOM OR WHAT DID YOU DEDICATE THIS CLASS?
(TURN TO PAGE 18 AND ADD YOUR ANSWER TO YOUR DEDICATION LOG.)

Notes and Takeaways

Self-Review

One a scale of 1 to 5 (low to high), rate the following areas of your performance during this session:

FOCUS: 1 2 3 4 5

EVENNESS OF BREATH: 1 2 3 4 5

BALANCE: 1 2 3 4 5

STRENGTH: 1 2 3 4 5

ENERGY LEVEL: 1 2 3 4 5

ATTITUDE: 1 2 3 4 5

Yoga Session (10)

DATE / / **TIME** -

☐ **Group Class Practice**

☐ **Home Practice and/or Private Instruction**

NAME OF STUDIO:

(OR) IN WHAT ROOM/SPACE DID YOU PRACTICE?

NAME OF TEACHER:

TEACHER RATING (CIRCLE ONE): A+ A A- B C D F

ON WHAT PART OF THE BODY DID YOU FOCUS DURING THIS SESSION?

CLASS LEVEL:
☐ BEGINNER ☐ INTERMEDIATE ☐ ADVANCED

☐ ABDOMINALS ☐ HIPS
☐ BACK ☐ BUTTOCKS

CROWD LEVEL: 1 2 3 4 5

☐ SHOULDERS ☐ LEGS

NOT CROWDED ▸ CROWDED

☐ ARMS ☐ ANKLES/FEET

TEMPERATURE: ☐ HEATED ☐ UNHEATED

☐ WRISTS/HANDS ☐ OTHER:

Session Details

WHAT STYLE DID YOU PRACTICE DURING THIS SESSION?

☐ ANUSARA	☐ KRIPALU
☐ ASHTANGA	☐ KUNDALINI
☐ BIKRAM	☐ POWER
☐ IYENGAR	☐ RESTORATIVE
☐ JIVAMUKTI	☐ VINIYOGA
	☐ OTHER:

WHAT TOOLS DID YOU HAVE ON HAND?

☐ MAT	☐ STRAP
☐ WATER BOTTLE	☐ BLANKET
☐ TOWEL	☐ BOLSTER PILLOW
☐ BLOCK	☐ OTHER:

SOUND ACCOMPANIMENT: ☐ NO MUSIC ☐ MUSIC

FAVORITE TRACK FROM TODAY'S SESSION
(TURN TO PAGE 20 AND ADD THE SONG TO YOUR YOGA SOUNDTRACK.)

Overall Session Rating

PACE OF FLOW: 1 2 3 4 5

FAVORITE POSE OF TODAY'S SESSION:

DYNAMISM OF SEQUENCING: 1 2 3 4 5

MOST CHALLENGING POSE:

DIFFICULTY: 1 2 3 4 5

POSES INCLUDED IN TODAY'S SEQUENCING:

POSE YOU HADN'T TRIED BEFORE TODAY:

☐ STANDING POSES	☐ FORWARD BENDS
☐ BALANCING POSES	☐ BACKBENDS
☐ SEATED POSES	☐ INVERSIONS
☐ ABDOMINAL STRENGTHENERS	☐ RESTING POSES
☐ TWISTS	

POSE IN WHICH YOU SHOWED THE MOST IMPROVEMENT:

POSE YOU'D LIKE TO WORK ON IN THE NEXT SESSION:

Dedication

TO WHOM OR WHAT DID YOU DEDICATE THIS CLASS?
(TURN TO PAGE 18 AND ADD YOUR ANSWER TO YOUR DEDICATION LOG.)

Notes and Takeaways

Self-Review

One a scale of 1 to 5 (low to high), rate the following areas of your performance during this session:

FOCUS:	1	2	3	4	5
EVENNESS OF BREATH:	1	2	3	4	5
BALANCE:	1	2	3	4	5
STRENGTH:	1	2	3	4	5
ENERGY LEVEL:	1	2	3	4	5
ATTITUDE:	1	2	3	4	5

DATE / / **TIME** -

☐ **Group Class Practice**

☐ **Home Practice and/or Private Instruction**

(OR)

NAME OF STUDIO:

IN WHAT ROOM/SPACE DID YOU PRACTICE?

NAME OF TEACHER:

TEACHER RATING (CIRCLE ONE): A+ A A- B C D F

CLASS LEVEL:

☐ BEGINNER ☐ INTERMEDIATE ☐ ADVANCED

CROWD LEVEL: ①②③④⑤
NOT CROWDED ▸ CROWDED

TEMPERATURE: ☐ HEATED ☐ UNHEATED

ON WHAT PART OF THE BODY DID YOU FOCUS DURING THIS SESSION?

☐ ABDOMINALS ☐ HIPS
☐ BACK ☐ BUTTOCKS
☐ SHOULDERS ☐ LEGS
☐ ARMS ☐ ANKLES/FEET
☐ WRISTS/HANDS ☐ OTHER:

Session Details

WHAT STYLE DID YOU PRACTICE DURING THIS SESSION?

☐ ANUSARA ☐ KRIPALU
☐ ASHTANGA ☐ KUNDALINI
☐ BIKRAM ☐ POWER
☐ IYENGAR ☐ RESTORATIVE
☐ JIVAMUKTI ☐ VINIYOGA
☐ OTHER:

WHAT TOOLS DID YOU HAVE ON HAND?

☐ MAT ☐ STRAP
☐ WATER BOTTLE ☐ BLANKET
☐ TOWEL ☐ BOLSTER PILLOW
☐ BLOCK ☐ OTHER:

SOUND ACCOMPANIMENT: ☐ NO MUSIC ☐ MUSIC

FAVORITE TRACK FROM TODAY'S SESSION
(TURN TO PAGE 20 AND ADD THE SONG TO YOUR YOGA SOUNDTRACK.)

Overall Session Rating

PACE OF FLOW: ①②③④⑤

DYNAMISM OF SEQUENCING: ①②③④⑤

DIFFICULTY: ①②③④⑤

POSES INCLUDED IN TODAY'S SEQUENCING:

☐ STANDING POSES ☐ FORWARD BENDS
☐ BALANCING POSES ☐ BACKBENDS
☐ SEATED POSES ☐ INVERSIONS
☐ ABDOMINAL STRENGTHENERS ☐ RESTING POSES
☐ TWISTS

FAVORITE POSE OF TODAY'S SESSION:

MOST CHALLENGING POSE:

POSE YOU HADN'T TRIED BEFORE TODAY:

POSE IN WHICH YOU SHOWED THE MOST IMPROVEMENT:

POSE YOU'D LIKE TO WORK ON IN THE NEXT SESSION:

Dedication

TO WHOM OR WHAT DID YOU DEDICATE THIS CLASS?
(TURN TO PAGE 18 AND ADD YOUR ANSWER TO YOUR DEDICATION LOG.)

Notes and Takeaways

Self-Review

One a scale of 1 to 5 (low to high), rate the following areas of your performance during this session:

FOCUS: 1 2 3 4 5

EVENNESS
OF BREATH: 1 2 3 4 5

BALANCE: 1 2 3 4 5

STRENGTH: 1 2 3 4 5

ENERGY
LEVEL: 1 2 3 4 5

ATTITUDE: 1 2 3 4 5

DATE   /   /   TIME   -

☐ **Group Class Practice**   ☐ **Home Practice and/or**
                                                  Private Instruction

NAME OF STUDIO: (OR)   IN WHAT ROOM/SPACE DID YOU PRACTICE?

NAME OF TEACHER:

TEACHER RATING (CIRCLE ONE): A+ A A- B C D F   ON WHAT PART OF THE BODY DID YOU FOCUS
                                                          DURING THIS SESSION?

CLASS LEVEL: ☐ ABDOMINALS   ☐ HIPS
☐ BEGINNER   ☐ INTERMEDIATE   ☐ ADVANCED   ☐ BACK   ☐ BUTTOCKS

CROWD LEVEL: 1 2 3 4 5   ☐ SHOULDERS   ☐ LEGS
        NOT CROWDED ▸ CROWDED   ☐ ARMS   ☐ ANKLES/FEET

TEMPERATURE: ☐ HEATED   ☐ UNHEATED   ☐ WRISTS/HANDS   ☐ OTHER:

Session Details

WHAT STYLE DID YOU PRACTICE DURING THIS SESSION?   WHAT TOOLS DID YOU HAVE ON HAND?

☐ ANUSARA   ☐ KRIPALU   ☐ MAT   ☐ STRAP
☐ ASHTANGA   ☐ KUNDALINI   ☐ WATER BOTTLE   ☐ BLANKET
☐ BIKRAM   ☐ POWER   ☐ TOWEL   ☐ BOLSTER PILLOW
☐ IYENGAR   ☐ RESTORATIVE   ☐ BLOCK   ☐ OTHER:
☐ JIVAMUKTI   ☐ VINIYOGA
                 ☐ OTHER:

SOUND ACCOMPANIMENT: ☐ NO MUSIC   ☐ MUSIC

FAVORITE TRACK FROM TODAY'S SESSION
(TURN TO PAGE 26 AND ADD THE SONG TO YOUR YOGA SOUNDTRACK.)

Overall Session Rating

PACE OF FLOW: 1 2 3 4 5   FAVORITE POSE OF TODAY'S SESSION:

DYNAMISM OF   1 2 3 4 5
SEQUENCING:
                                        MOST CHALLENGING POSE:
DIFFICULTY: 1 2 3 4 5

POSES INCLUDED IN TODAY'S SEQUENCING: POSE YOU HADN'T TRIED BEFORE TODAY:

☐ STANDING POSES   ☐ FORWARD BENDS
☐ BALANCING POSES   ☐ BACKBENDS   POSE IN WHICH YOU SHOWED THE MOST IMPROVEMENT:
☐ SEATED POSES   ☐ INVERSIONS
☐ ABDOMINAL   ☐ RESTING POSES
  STRENGTHENERS   POSE YOU'D LIKE TO WORK ON IN THE NEXT SESSION:
☐ TWISTS

Dedication

TO WHOM OR WHAT DID YOU DEDICATE THIS CLASS?
(TURN TO PAGE 18 AND ADD YOUR ANSWER TO YOUR DEDICATION LOG.)

Notes and Takeaways

Self-Review

One a scale of 1 to 5 (low to high), rate the following areas of your performance during this session:

FOCUS: 1 2 3 4 5

EVENNESS OF BREATH: 1 2 3 4 5

BALANCE: 1 2 3 4 5

STRENGTH: 1 2 3 4 5

ENERGY LEVEL: 1 2 3 4 5

ATTITUDE: 1 2 3 4 5

DATE   /   /   TIME   -

☐ **Group Class Practice**

☐ **Home Practice and/or Private Instruction**

(OR)

NAME OF STUDIO:

IN WHAT ROOM/SPACE DID YOU PRACTICE?

NAME OF TEACHER:

TEACHER RATING (CIRCLE ONE): A+ A A- B C D F

CLASS LEVEL:

☐ BEGINNER ☐ INTERMEDIATE ☐ ADVANCED

CROWD LEVEL: ① ② ③ ④ ⑤

NOT CROWDED ▸ CROWDED

TEMPERATURE: ☐ HEATED ☐ UNHEATED

ON WHAT PART OF THE BODY DID YOU FOCUS DURING THIS SESSION?

☐ ABDOMINALS   ☐ HIPS
☐ BACK   ☐ BUTTOCKS
☐ SHOULDERS   ☐ LEGS
☐ ARMS   ☐ ANKLES/FEET
☐ WRISTS/HANDS   ☐ OTHER:

Session Details

WHAT STYLE DID YOU PRACTICE DURING THIS SESSION?

☐ ANUSARA   ☐ KRIPALU
☐ ASHTANGA   ☐ KUNDALINI
☐ BIKRAM   ☐ POWER
☐ IYENGAR   ☐ RESTORATIVE
☐ JIVAMUKTI   ☐ VINIYOGA
                   ☐ OTHER:

WHAT TOOLS DID YOU HAVE ON HAND?

☐ MAT   ☐ STRAP
☐ WATER BOTTLE   ☐ BLANKET
☐ TOWEL   ☐ BOLSTER PILLOW
☐ BLOCK   ☐ OTHER:

SOUND ACCOMPANIMENT: ☐ NO MUSIC ☐ MUSIC

FAVORITE TRACK FROM TODAY'S SESSION
(TURN TO PAGE 20 AND ADD THE SONG TO YOUR YOGA SOUNDTRACK.)

Overall Session Rating

PACE OF FLOW: ① ② ③ ④ ⑤

DYNAMISM OF SEQUENCING: ① ② ③ ④ ⑤

DIFFICULTY: ① ② ③ ④ ⑤

POSES INCLUDED IN TODAY'S SEQUENCING:

☐ STANDING POSES   ☐ FORWARD BENDS
☐ BALANCING POSES   ☐ BACKBENDS
☐ SEATED POSES   ☐ INVERSIONS
☐ ABDOMINAL   ☐ RESTING POSES
  STRENGTHENERS
☐ TWISTS

FAVORITE POSE OF TODAY'S SESSION:

MOST CHALLENGING POSE:

POSE YOU HADN'T TRIED BEFORE TODAY:

POSE IN WHICH YOU SHOWED THE MOST IMPROVEMENT:

POSE YOU'D LIKE TO WORK ON IN THE NEXT SESSION:

Dedication

TO WHOM OR WHAT DID YOU DEDICATE THIS CLASS?
(TURN TO PAGE 18 AND ADD YOUR ANSWER TO YOUR DEDICATION LOG.)

Notes and Takeaways

Self-Review

One a scale of 1 to 5 (low to high), rate the following areas of your performance during this session:

FOCUS: ①-②-③-④-⑤

EVENNESS
OF BREATH: ①-②-③-④-⑤

BALANCE: ①-②-③-④-⑤

STRENGTH: ①-②-③-④-⑤

ENERGY
LEVEL: ①-②-③-④-⑤

ATTITUDE: ①-②-③-④-⑤

DATE   /   /   TIME   -

☐ **Group Class Practice**

☐ **Home Practice and/or Private Instruction**

NAME OF STUDIO: (OR)   IN WHAT ROOM/SPACE DID YOU PRACTICE?

NAME OF TEACHER:

TEACHER RATING (CIRCLE ONE): A+ A A- B C D F

CLASS LEVEL:
☐ BEGINNER ☐ INTERMEDIATE ☐ ADVANCED

CROWD LEVEL: ① ② ③ ④ ⑤
        NOT CROWDED ▸ CROWDED

TEMPERATURE: ☐ HEATED   ☐ UNHEATED

ON WHAT PART OF THE BODY DID YOU FOCUS DURING THIS SESSION?
☐ ABDOMINALS   ☐ HIPS
☐ BACK   ☐ BUTTOCKS
☐ SHOULDERS   ☐ LEGS
☐ ARMS   ☐ ANKLES/FEET
☐ WRISTS/HANDS ☐ OTHER:

Session Details

WHAT STYLE DID YOU PRACTICE DURING THIS SESSION?
☐ ANUSARA   ☐ KRIPALU
☐ ASHTANGA   ☐ KUNDALINI
☐ BIKRAM   ☐ POWER
☐ IYENGAR   ☐ RESTORATIVE
☐ JIVAMUKTI   ☐ VINIYOGA
                ☐ OTHER:

WHAT TOOLS DID YOU HAVE ON HAND?
☐ MAT   ☐ STRAP
☐ WATER BOTTLE   ☐ BLANKET
☐ TOWEL   ☐ BOLSTER PILLOW
☐ BLOCK   ☐ OTHER:

SOUND ACCOMPANIMENT: ☐ NO MUSIC   ☐ MUSIC

FAVORITE TRACK FROM TODAY'S SESSION
(TURN TO PAGE 20 AND ADD THE SONG TO YOUR YOGA SOUNDTRACK.)

Overall Session Rating

PACE OF FLOW: ① ② ③ ④ ⑤

DYNAMISM OF SEQUENCING: ① ② ③ ④ ⑤

DIFFICULTY: ① ② ③ ④ ⑤

POSES INCLUDED IN TODAY'S SEQUENCING:
☐ STANDING POSES   ☐ FORWARD BENDS
☐ BALANCING POSES   ☐ BACKBENDS
☐ SEATED POSES   ☐ INVERSIONS
☐ ABDOMINAL STRENGTHENERS   ☐ RESTING POSES
☐ TWISTS

FAVORITE POSE OF TODAY'S SESSION:

MOST CHALLENGING POSE:

POSE YOU HADN'T TRIED BEFORE TODAY:

POSE IN WHICH YOU SHOWED THE MOST IMPROVEMENT:

POSE YOU'D LIKE TO WORK ON IN THE NEXT SESSION:

Dedication

TO WHOM OR WHAT DID YOU DEDICATE THIS CLASS?
(TURN TO PAGE 18 AND ADD YOUR ANSWER TO YOUR DEDICATION LOG.)

Notes and Takeaways

Self-Review

One a scale of 1 to 5 (low to high), rate the following areas of your performance during this session:

FOCUS: 1 2 3 4 5

EVENNESS OF BREATH: 1 2 3 4 5

BALANCE: 1 2 3 4 5

STRENGTH: 1 2 3 4 5

ENERGY LEVEL: 1 2 3 4 5

ATTITUDE: 1 2 3 4 5

DATE / / **TIME** -

☐ **Group Class Practice** (OR) ☐ **Home Practice and/or Private Instruction**

NAME OF STUDIO:

IN WHAT ROOM/SPACE DID YOU PRACTICE?

NAME OF TEACHER:

TEACHER RATING (CIRCLE ONE): A+ A A- B C D F

ON WHAT PART OF THE BODY DID YOU FOCUS DURING THIS SESSION?

CLASS LEVEL:
☐ BEGINNER ☐ INTERMEDIATE ☐ ADVANCED

☐ ABDOMINALS ☐ HIPS
☐ BACK ☐ BUTTOCKS

CROWD LEVEL: (1) (2) (3) (4) (5)
NOT CROWDED ▸ CROWDED

☐ SHOULDERS ☐ LEGS
☐ ARMS ☐ ANKLES/FEET

TEMPERATURE: ☐ HEATED ☐ UNHEATED

☐ WRISTS/HANDS ☐ OTHER:

Session Details

WHAT STYLE DID YOU PRACTICE DURING THIS SESSION?

☐ ANUSARA ☐ KRIPALU
☐ ASHTANGA ☐ KUNDALINI
☐ BIKRAM ☐ POWER
☐ IYENGAR ☐ RESTORATIVE
☐ JIVAMUKTI ☐ VINIYOGA
☐ OTHER:

WHAT TOOLS DID YOU HAVE ON HAND?
☐ MAT ☐ STRAP
☐ WATER BOTTLE ☐ BLANKET
☐ TOWEL ☐ BOLSTER PILLOW
☐ BLOCK ☐ OTHER:

SOUND ACCOMPANIMENT: ☐ NO MUSIC ☐ MUSIC

FAVORITE TRACK FROM TODAY'S SESSION
(TURN TO PAGE 20 AND ADD THE SONG TO YOUR YOGA SOUNDTRACK.)

Overall Session Rating

PACE OF FLOW: (1) (2) (3) (4) (5)

DYNAMISM OF SEQUENCING: (1) (2) (3) (4) (5)

DIFFICULTY: (1) (2) (3) (4) (5)

FAVORITE POSE OF TODAY'S SESSION:

MOST CHALLENGING POSE:

POSES INCLUDED IN TODAY'S SEQUENCING:

☐ STANDING POSES ☐ FORWARD BENDS
☐ BALANCING POSES ☐ BACKBENDS
☐ SEATED POSES ☐ INVERSIONS
☐ ABDOMINAL STRENGTHENERS ☐ RESTING POSES
☐ TWISTS

POSE YOU HADN'T TRIED BEFORE TODAY:

POSE IN WHICH YOU SHOWED THE MOST IMPROVEMENT:

POSE YOU'D LIKE TO WORK ON IN THE NEXT SESSION:

Dedication

TO WHOM OR WHAT DID YOU DEDICATE THIS CLASS?
(TURN TO PAGE 18 AND ADD YOUR ANSWER TO YOUR DEDICATION LOG.)

Notes and Takeaways

Self-Review

One a scale of 1 to 5 (low to high), rate the following areas of your performance during this session:

FOCUS: ① ② ③ ④ ⑤

EVENNESS OF BREATH: ① ② ③ ④ ⑤

BALANCE: ① ② ③ ④ ⑤

STRENGTH: ① ② ③ ④ ⑤

ENERGY LEVEL: ① ② ③ ④ ⑤

ATTITUDE: ① ② ③ ④ ⑤

DATE / / **TIME** -

☐ **Group Class Practice**

☐ **Home Practice and/or Private Instruction**

(OR)

NAME OF STUDIO:

IN WHAT ROOM/SPACE DID YOU PRACTICE?

NAME OF TEACHER:

TEACHER RATING (CIRCLE ONE): A+ A A- B C D F

ON WHAT PART OF THE BODY DID YOU FOCUS DURING THIS SESSION?

CLASS LEVEL:

☐ BEGINNER ☐ INTERMEDIATE ☐ ADVANCED

CROWD LEVEL: 1 2 3 4 5

NOT CROWDED ▸ CROWDED

TEMPERATURE: ☐ HEATED ☐ UNHEATED

☐ ABDOMINALS ☐ HIPS
☐ BACK ☐ BUTTOCKS
☐ SHOULDERS ☐ LEGS
☐ ARMS ☐ ANKLES/FEET
☐ WRISTS/HANDS ☐ OTHER:

Session Details

WHAT STYLE DID YOU PRACTICE DURING THIS SESSION?

☐ ANUSARA ☐ KRIPALU
☐ ASHTANGA ☐ KUNDALINI
☐ BIKRAM ☐ POWER
☐ IYENGAR ☐ RESTORATIVE
☐ JIVAMUKTI ☐ VINIYOGA
☐ OTHER:

WHAT TOOLS DID YOU HAVE ON HAND?

☐ MAT ☐ STRAP
☐ WATER BOTTLE ☐ BLANKET
☐ TOWEL ☐ BOLSTER PILLOW
☐ BLOCK ☐ OTHER:

SOUND ACCOMPANIMENT: ☐ NO MUSIC ☐ MUSIC

FAVORITE TRACK FROM TODAY'S SESSION
(TURN TO PAGE 20 AND ADD THE SONG TO YOUR YOGA SOUNDTRACK.)

Overall Session Rating

PACE OF FLOW: 1 2 3 4 5

DYNAMISM OF SEQUENCING: 1 2 3 4 5

DIFFICULTY: 1 2 3 4 5

FAVORITE POSE OF TODAY'S SESSION:

MOST CHALLENGING POSE:

POSES INCLUDED IN TODAY'S SEQUENCING:

☐ STANDING POSES ☐ FORWARD BENDS
☐ BALANCING POSES ☐ BACKBENDS
☐ SEATED POSES ☐ INVERSIONS
☐ ABDOMINAL STRENGTHENERS ☐ RESTING POSES
☐ TWISTS

POSE YOU HADN'T TRIED BEFORE TODAY:

POSE IN WHICH YOU SHOWED THE MOST IMPROVEMENT:

POSE YOU'D LIKE TO WORK ON IN THE NEXT SESSION:

Dedication

TO WHOM OR WHAT DID YOU DEDICATE THIS CLASS?
(TURN TO PAGE 18 AND ADD YOUR ANSWER TO YOUR DEDICATION LOG.)

Notes and Takeaways

Self-Review

One a scale of 1 to 5 (low to high), rate the following areas of your performance during this session:

FOCUS: 1 2 3 4 5

EVENNESS
OF BREATH: 1 2 3 4 5

BALANCE: 1 2 3 4 5

STRENGTH: 1 2 3 4 5

ENERGY
LEVEL: 1 2 3 4 5

ATTITUDE: 1 2 3 4 5

Yoga Session 17

DATE   /   /   **TIME**   -

☐ **Group Class Practice**

☐ **Home Practice and/or Private Instruction**

OR

NAME OF STUDIO:

IN WHAT ROOM/SPACE DID YOU PRACTICE?

NAME OF TEACHER:

TEACHER RATING (CIRCLE ONE): A+ A A- B C D F

CLASS LEVEL:
☐ BEGINNER ☐ INTERMEDIATE ☐ ADVANCED

CROWD LEVEL: 1 2 3 4 5
NOT CROWDED ▸ CROWDED

TEMPERATURE: ☐ HEATED ☐ UNHEATED

ON WHAT PART OF THE BODY DID YOU FOCUS DURING THIS SESSION?
☐ ABDOMINALS ☐ HIPS
☐ BACK ☐ BUTTOCKS
☐ SHOULDERS ☐ LEGS
☐ ARMS ☐ ANKLES/FEET
☐ WRISTS/HANDS ☐ OTHER:

Session Details

WHAT STYLE DID YOU PRACTICE DURING THIS SESSION?
☐ ANUSARA ☐ KRIPALU
☐ ASHTANGA ☐ KUNDALINI
☐ BIKRAM ☐ POWER
☐ IYENGAR ☐ RESTORATIVE
☐ JIVAMUKTI ☐ VINIYOGA
☐ OTHER:

WHAT TOOLS DID YOU HAVE ON HAND?
☐ MAT ☐ STRAP
☐ WATER BOTTLE ☐ BLANKET
☐ TOWEL ☐ BOLSTER PILLOW
☐ BLOCK ☐ OTHER:

SOUND ACCOMPANIMENT: ☐ NO MUSIC ☐ MUSIC

FAVORITE TRACK FROM TODAY'S SESSION
(TURN TO PAGE 20 AND ADD THE SONG TO YOUR YOGA SOUNDTRACK.)

Overall Session Rating

PACE OF FLOW: 1 2 3 4 5

DYNAMISM OF SEQUENCING: 1 2 3 4 5

DIFFICULTY: 1 2 3 4 5

POSES INCLUDED IN TODAY'S SEQUENCING:
☐ STANDING POSES ☐ FORWARD BENDS
☐ BALANCING POSES ☐ BACKBENDS
☐ SEATED POSES ☐ INVERSIONS
☐ ABDOMINAL STRENGTHENERS ☐ RESTING POSES
☐ TWISTS

FAVORITE POSE OF TODAY'S SESSION:

MOST CHALLENGING POSE:

POSE YOU HADN'T TRIED BEFORE TODAY:

POSE IN WHICH YOU SHOWED THE MOST IMPROVEMENT:

POSE YOU'D LIKE TO WORK ON IN THE NEXT SESSION:

Dedication

TO WHOM OR WHAT DID YOU DEDICATE THIS CLASS?
(TURN TO PAGE 18 AND ADD YOUR ANSWER TO YOUR DEDICATION LOG.)

Notes and Takeaways

Self-Review

One a scale of 1 to 5 (low to high), rate the following areas of your performance during this session:

FOCUS:	1	2	3	4	5
EVENNESS OF BREATH:	1	2	3	4	5
BALANCE:	1	2	3	4	5
STRENGTH:	1	2	3	4	5
ENERGY LEVEL:	1	2	3	4	5
ATTITUDE:	1	2	3	4	5

DATE / / **TIME** -

☐ Group Class Practice

NAME OF STUDIO:

NAME OF TEACHER:

TEACHER RATING (CIRCLE ONE): A+ A A- B C D F

CLASS LEVEL:
☐ BEGINNER ☐ INTERMEDIATE ☐ ADVANCED

CROWD LEVEL: 1 2 3 4 5
NOT CROWDED ▸ CROWDED

TEMPERATURE: ☐ HEATED ☐ UNHEATED

(OR)

☐ Home Practice and/or Private Instruction

IN WHAT ROOM/SPACE DID YOU PRACTICE?

ON WHAT PART OF THE BODY DID YOU FOCUS DURING THIS SESSION?

☐ ABDOMINALS   ☐ HIPS
☐ BACK   ☐ BUTTOCKS
☐ SHOULDERS   ☐ LEGS
☐ ARMS   ☐ ANKLES/FEET
☐ WRISTS/HANDS   ☐ OTHER:

Session Details

WHAT STYLE DID YOU PRACTICE DURING THIS SESSION?

☐ ANUSARA   ☐ KRIPALU
☐ ASHTANGA   ☐ KUNDALINI
☐ BIKRAM   ☐ POWER
☐ IYENGAR   ☐ RESTORATIVE
☐ JIVAMUKTI   ☐ VINIYOGA
               ☐ OTHER:

WHAT TOOLS DID YOU HAVE ON HAND?

☐ MAT   ☐ STRAP
☐ WATER BOTTLE   ☐ BLANKET
☐ TOWEL   ☐ BOLSTER PILLOW
☐ BLOCK   ☐ OTHER:

SOUND ACCOMPANIMENT: ☐ NO MUSIC ☐ MUSIC

FAVORITE TRACK FROM TODAY'S SESSION
(TURN TO PAGE 20 AND ADD THE SONG TO YOUR YOGA SOUNDTRACK.)

Overall Session Rating

PACE OF FLOW: 1 2 3 4 5

DYNAMISM OF SEQUENCING: 1 2 3 4 5

DIFFICULTY: 1 2 3 4 5

POSES INCLUDED IN TODAY'S SEQUENCING:

☐ STANDING POSES   ☐ FORWARD BENDS
☐ BALANCING POSES   ☐ BACKBENDS
☐ SEATED POSES   ☐ INVERSIONS
☐ ABDOMINAL STRENGTHENERS   ☐ RESTING POSES
☐ TWISTS

FAVORITE POSE OF TODAY'S SESSION:

MOST CHALLENGING POSE:

POSE YOU HADN'T TRIED BEFORE TODAY:

POSE IN WHICH YOU SHOWED THE MOST IMPROVEMENT:

POSE YOU'D LIKE TO WORK ON IN THE NEXT SESSION:

Dedication

TO WHOM OR WHAT DID YOU DEDICATE THIS CLASS?
(TURN TO PAGE 18 AND ADD YOUR ANSWER TO YOUR DEDICATION LOG.)

Notes and Takeaways

Self-Review

One a scale of 1 to 5 (low to high), rate the following areas of your performance during this session:

FOCUS: 1 2 3 4 5

EVENNESS
OF BREATH: 1 2 3 4 5

BALANCE: 1 2 3 4 5

STRENGTH: 1 2 3 4 5

ENERGY
LEVEL: 1 2 3 4 5

ATTITUDE: 1 2 3 4 5

Yoga Session (19)

DATE   /   /   TIME   -

☐ **Group Class Practice**   ☐ **Home Practice and/or Private Instruction**

NAME OF STUDIO: (OR)   IN WHAT ROOM/SPACE DID YOU PRACTICE?

NAME OF TEACHER:

TEACHER RATING (CIRCLE ONE): A+ A A- B C D F   ON WHAT PART OF THE BODY DID YOU FOCUS DURING THIS SESSION?

CLASS LEVEL:
☐ BEGINNER   ☐ INTERMEDIATE   ☐ ADVANCED   ☐ ABDOMINALS   ☐ HIPS
                                                 ☐ BACK   ☐ BUTTOCKS
CROWD LEVEL: 1 2 3 4 5   ☐ SHOULDERS   ☐ LEGS
          NOT CROWDED ▸ CROWDED   ☐ ARMS   ☐ ANKLES/FEET
TEMPERATURE: ☐ HEATED   ☐ UNHEATED   ☐ WRISTS/HANDS   ☐ OTHER:

Session Details

WHAT STYLE DID YOU PRACTICE DURING THIS SESSION?   WHAT TOOLS DID YOU HAVE ON HAND?
☐ ANUSARA   ☐ KRIPALU   ☐ MAT   ☐ STRAP
☐ ASHTANGA   ☐ KUNDALINI   ☐ WATER BOTTLE   ☐ BLANKET
☐ BIKRAM   ☐ POWER   ☐ TOWEL   ☐ BOLSTER PILLOW
☐ IYENGAR   ☐ RESTORATIVE   ☐ BLOCK   ☐ OTHER:
☐ JIVAMUKTI   ☐ VINIYOGA
                 ☐ OTHER:

SOUND ACCOMPANIMENT: ☐ NO MUSIC   ☐ MUSIC

FAVORITE TRACK FROM TODAY'S SESSION
TURN TO PAGE 23 AND ADD THE SONG TO YOUR YOGA SOUNDTRACK

Overall Session Rating

PACE OF FLOW: 1 2 3 4 5   FAVORITE POSE OF TODAY'S SESSION:

DYNAMISM OF
SEQUENCING: 1 2 3 4 5   MOST CHALLENGING POSE:

DIFFICULTY: 1 2 3 4 5
                                         POSE YOU HADN'T TRIED BEFORE TODAY:
POSES INCLUDED IN TODAY'S SEQUENCING:
☐ STANDING POSES   ☐ FORWARD BENDS
☐ BALANCING POSES   ☐ BACKBENDS   POSE IN WHICH YOU SHOWED THE MOST IMPROVEMENT:
☐ SEATED POSES   ☐ INVERSIONS
☐ ABDOMINAL   ☐ RESTING POSES
  STRENGTHENERS   POSE YOU'D LIKE TO WORK ON IN THE NEXT SESSION:
☐ TWISTS

Dedication

TO WHOM OR WHAT DID YOU DEDICATE THIS CLASS?
(TURN TO PAGE 18 AND ADD YOUR ANSWER TO YOUR DEDICATION LOG.)

Notes and Takeaways

Self-Review

One a scale of 1 to 5 (low to high), rate the following areas of your performance during this session:

FOCUS: 1 2 3 4 5

EVENNESS OF BREATH: 1 2 3 4 5

BALANCE: 1 2 3 4 5

STRENGTH: 1 2 3 4 5

ENERGY LEVEL: 1 2 3 4 5

ATTITUDE: 1 2 3 4 5

DATE   /   /   TIME   -

☐ **Group Class Practice**

☐ **Home Practice and/or Private Instruction**

(OR)

NAME OF STUDIO: **IN WHAT ROOM/SPACE DID YOU PRACTICE?**

NAME OF TEACHER:

TEACHER RATING (CIRCLE ONE): A+ A A- B C D F

CLASS LEVEL:

☐ BEGINNER   ☐ INTERMEDIATE   ☐ ADVANCED

CROWD LEVEL: (1) (2) (3) (4) (5)

        NOT CROWDED ▸ CROWDED

TEMPERATURE: ☐ HEATED   ☐ UNHEATED

ON WHAT PART OF THE BODY DID YOU FOCUS DURING THIS SESSION?

☐ ABDOMINALS   ☐ HIPS
☐ BACK   ☐ BUTTOCKS
☐ SHOULDERS   ☐ LEGS
☐ ARMS   ☐ ANKLES/FEET
☐ WRISTS/HANDS   ☐ OTHER:

Session Details

WHAT STYLE DID YOU PRACTICE DURING THIS SESSION?

☐ ANUSARA   ☐ KRIPALU
☐ ASHTANGA   ☐ KUNDALINI
☐ BIKRAM   ☐ POWER
☐ IYENGAR   ☐ RESTORATIVE
☐ JIVAMUKTI   ☐ VINIYOGA
               ☐ OTHER:

WHAT TOOLS DID YOU HAVE ON HAND?

☐ MAT   ☐ STRAP
☐ WATER BOTTLE   ☐ BLANKET
☐ TOWEL   ☐ BOLSTER PILLOW
☐ BLOCK   ☐ OTHER:

SOUND ACCOMPANIMENT: ☐ NO MUSIC   ☐ MUSIC

FAVORITE TRACK FROM TODAY'S SESSION
[TURN TO PAGE 20 AND ADD THE SONG TO YOUR YOGA SOUNDTRACK.]

Overall Session Rating

PACE OF FLOW: 1 2 3 4 5

DYNAMISM OF SEQUENCING: 1 2 3 4 5

DIFFICULTY: 1 2 3 4 5

POSES INCLUDED IN TODAY'S SEQUENCING:

☐ STANDING POSES   ☐ FORWARD BENDS
☐ BALANCING POSES   ☐ BACKBENDS
☐ SEATED POSES   ☐ INVERSIONS
☐ ABDOMINAL STRENGTHENERS   ☐ RESTING POSES
☐ TWISTS

FAVORITE POSE OF TODAY'S SESSION:

MOST CHALLENGING POSE:

POSE YOU HADN'T TRIED BEFORE TODAY:

POSE IN WHICH YOU SHOWED THE MOST IMPROVEMENT:

POSE YOU'D LIKE TO WORK ON IN THE NEXT SESSION:

Dedication

TO WHOM OR WHAT DID YOU DEDICATE THIS CLASS?
(TURN TO PAGE 18 AND ADD YOUR ANSWER TO YOUR DEDICATION LOG.)

Notes and Takeaways

Self-Review

One a scale of 1 to 5 (low to high), rate the following areas of your performance during this session:

FOCUS: ①-②-③-④-⑤

EVENNESS OF BREATH: ①-②-③-④-⑤

BALANCE: ①-②-③-④-⑤

STRENGTH: ①-②-③-④-⑤

ENERGY LEVEL: ①-②-③-④-⑤

ATTITUDE: ①-②-③-④-⑤

DATE   /   /   TIME   -

☐ **Group Class Practice**

☐ **Home Practice and/or Private Instruction**

(OR)

NAME OF STUDIO:

IN WHAT ROOM/SPACE DID YOU PRACTICE?

NAME OF TEACHER:

TEACHER RATING (CIRCLE ONE): A+ A A- B C D F

ON WHAT PART OF THE BODY DID YOU FOCUS DURING THIS SESSION?

CLASS LEVEL:

☐ BEGINNER ☐ INTERMEDIATE ☐ ADVANCED

☐ ABDOMINALS   ☐ HIPS
☐ BACK   ☐ BUTTOCKS

CROWD LEVEL: ① ② ③ ④ ⑤

☐ SHOULDERS   ☐ LEGS

NOT CROWDED ▸ CROWDED

☐ ARMS   ☐ ANKLES/FEET

TEMPERATURE: ☐ HEATED ☐ UNHEATED

☐ WRISTS/HANDS   ☐ OTHER:

Session Details

WHAT STYLE DID YOU PRACTICE DURING THIS SESSION?

☐ ANUSARA	☐ KRIPALU
☐ ASHTANGA	☐ KUNDALINI
☐ BIKRAM	☐ POWER
☐ IYENGAR	☐ RESTORATIVE
☐ JIVAMUKTI	☐ VINIYOGA
	☐ OTHER:

WHAT TOOLS DID YOU HAVE ON HAND?

☐ MAT	☐ STRAP
☐ WATER BOTTLE	☐ BLANKET
☐ TOWEL	☐ BOLSTER PILLOW
☐ BLOCK	☐ OTHER:

SOUND ACCOMPANIMENT: ☐ NO MUSIC ☐ MUSIC

FAVORITE TRACK FROM TODAY'S SESSION
(TURN TO PAGE 20 AND ADD THE SONG TO YOUR YOGA SOUNDTRACK.)

Overall Session Rating

PACE OF FLOW: ① ② ③ ④ ⑤

FAVORITE POSE OF TODAY'S SESSION:

DYNAMISM OF SEQUENCING: ① ② ③ ④ ⑤

MOST CHALLENGING POSE:

DIFFICULTY: ① ② ③ ④ ⑤

POSES INCLUDED IN TODAY'S SEQUENCING:

POSE YOU HADN'T TRIED BEFORE TODAY:

☐ STANDING POSES	☐ FORWARD BENDS
☐ BALANCING POSES	☐ BACKBENDS
☐ SEATED POSES	☐ INVERSIONS
☐ ABDOMINAL STRENGTHENERS	☐ RESTING POSES
☐ TWISTS	

POSE IN WHICH YOU SHOWED THE MOST IMPROVEMENT:

POSE YOU'D LIKE TO WORK ON IN THE NEXT SESSION:

Dedication

TO WHOM OR WHAT DID YOU DEDICATE THIS CLASS?
(TURN TO PAGE 18 AND ADD YOUR ANSWER TO YOUR DEDICATION LOG.)

Notes and Takeaways

Self-Review

One a scale of 1 to 5 (low to high), rate the following areas of your performance during this session:

FOCUS: 1 2 3 4 5

EVENNESS OF BREATH: 1 2 3 4 5

BALANCE: 1 2 3 4 5

STRENGTH: 1 2 3 4 5

ENERGY LEVEL: 1 2 3 4 5

ATTITUDE: 1 2 3 4 5

DATE / /   **TIME** -

☐ **Group Class Practice**   ☐ **Home Practice and/or Private Instruction**

NAME OF STUDIO: _____   (OR)   **IN WHAT ROOM/SPACE DID YOU PRACTICE?**

NAME OF TEACHER: _____

TEACHER RATING (CIRCLE ONE): A+ A A- B C D F

CLASS LEVEL:
☐ BEGINNER ☐ INTERMEDIATE ☐ ADVANCED

CROWD LEVEL: (1)-(2)-(3)-(4)-(5)
            NOT CROWDED ▸ CROWDED

TEMPERATURE: ☐ HEATED   ☐ UNHEATED

ON WHAT PART OF THE BODY DID YOU FOCUS DURING THIS SESSION?
☐ ABDOMINALS   ☐ HIPS
☐ BACK   ☐ BUTTOCKS
☐ SHOULDERS   ☐ LEGS
☐ ARMS   ☐ ANKLES/FEET
☐ WRISTS/HANDS   ☐ OTHER: _____

Session Details

WHAT STYLE DID YOU PRACTICE DURING THIS SESSION?
☐ ANUSARA   ☐ KRIPALU
☐ ASHTANGA   ☐ KUNDALINI
☐ BIKRAM   ☐ POWER
☐ IYENGAR   ☐ RESTORATIVE
☐ JIVAMUKTI   ☐ VINIYOGA
                 ☐ OTHER: _____

WHAT TOOLS DID YOU HAVE ON HAND?
☐ MAT   ☐ STRAP
☐ WATER BOTTLE   ☐ BLANKET
☐ TOWEL   ☐ BOLSTER PILLOW
☐ BLOCK   ☐ OTHER: _____

SOUND ACCOMPANIMENT: ☐ NO MUSIC   ☐ MUSIC

FAVORITE TRACK FROM TODAY'S SESSION _____
(TURN TO PAGE 20 AND ADD THE SONG TO YOUR YOGA SOUNDTRACK.)

Overall Session Rating

PACE OF FLOW: (1)-(2)-(3)-(4)-(5)

DYNAMISM OF SEQUENCING: (1)-(2)-(3)-(4)-(5)

DIFFICULTY: (1)-(2)-(3)-(4)-(5)

POSES INCLUDED IN TODAY'S SEQUENCING:
☐ STANDING POSES   ☐ FORWARD BENDS
☐ BALANCING POSES   ☐ BACKBENDS
☐ SEATED POSES   ☐ INVERSIONS
☐ ABDOMINAL STRENGTHENERS   ☐ RESTING POSES
☐ TWISTS

FAVORITE POSE OF TODAY'S SESSION:

MOST CHALLENGING POSE:

POSE YOU HADN'T TRIED BEFORE TODAY:

POSE IN WHICH YOU SHOWED THE MOST IMPROVEMENT:

POSE YOU'D LIKE TO WORK ON IN THE NEXT SESSION:

Dedication

TO WHOM OR WHAT DID YOU DEDICATE THIS CLASS?
(TURN TO PAGE 18 AND ADD YOUR ANSWER TO YOUR DEDICATION LOG.)

Notes and Takeaways

Self-Review

One a scale of 1 to 5 (low to high), rate the following areas of your performance during this session:

FOCUS: 1 2 3 4 5

EVENNESS OF BREATH: 1 2 3 4 5

BALANCE: 1 2 3 4 5

STRENGTH: 1 2 3 4 5

ENERGY LEVEL: 1 2 3 4 5

ATTITUDE: 1 2 3 4 5

DATE   /   /   TIME   -

☐ **Group Class Practice**

NAME OF STUDIO:

NAME OF TEACHER:

TEACHER RATING (CIRCLE ONE): A+ A A- B C D F

CLASS LEVEL:
☐ BEGINNER   ☐ INTERMEDIATE   ☐ ADVANCED

CROWD LEVEL: ① ② ③ ④ ⑤
NOT CROWDED ▶ CROWDED

TEMPERATURE: ☐ HEATED   ☐ UNHEATED

(OR)

☐ **Home Practice and/or Private Instruction**

IN WHAT ROOM/SPACE DID YOU PRACTICE?

ON WHAT PART OF THE BODY DID YOU FOCUS DURING THIS SESSION?
☐ ABDOMINALS   ☐ HIPS
☐ BACK   ☐ BUTTOCKS
☐ SHOULDERS   ☐ LEGS
☐ ARMS   ☐ ANKLES/FEET
☐ WRISTS/HANDS   ☐ OTHER:

Session Details

WHAT STYLE DID YOU PRACTICE DURING THIS SESSION?
☐ ANUSARA   ☐ KRIPALU
☐ ASHTANGA   ☐ KUNDALINI
☐ BIKRAM   ☐ POWER
☐ IYENGAR   ☐ RESTORATIVE
☐ JIVAMUKTI   ☐ VINIYOGA
                 ☐ OTHER:

WHAT TOOLS DID YOU HAVE ON HAND?
☐ MAT   ☐ STRAP
☐ WATER BOTTLE   ☐ BLANKET
☐ TOWEL   ☐ BOLSTER PILLOW
☐ BLOCK   ☐ OTHER:

SOUND ACCOMPANIMENT: ☐ NO MUSIC   ☐ MUSIC

FAVORITE TRACK FROM TODAY'S SESSION
(TURN TO PAGE 20 AND ADD THE SONG TO YOUR YOGA SOUNDTRACK.)

Overall Session Rating

PACE OF FLOW: ① ② ③ ④ ⑤

DYNAMISM OF SEQUENCING: ① ② ③ ④ ⑤

DIFFICULTY: ① ② ③ ④ ⑤

POSES INCLUDED IN TODAY'S SEQUENCING:
☐ STANDING POSES   ☐ FORWARD BENDS
☐ BALANCING POSES   ☐ BACKBENDS
☐ SEATED POSES   ☐ INVERSIONS
☐ ABDOMINAL STRENGTHENERS   ☐ RESTING POSES
☐ TWISTS

FAVORITE POSE OF TODAY'S SESSION:

MOST CHALLENGING POSE:

POSE YOU HADN'T TRIED BEFORE TODAY:

POSE IN WHICH YOU SHOWED THE MOST IMPROVEMENT:

POSE YOU'D LIKE TO WORK ON IN THE NEXT SESSION:

Dedication

TO WHOM OR WHAT DID YOU DEDICATE THIS CLASS?
(TURN TO PAGE 18 AND ADD YOUR ANSWER TO YOUR DEDICATION LOG.)

Notes and Takeaways

Self-Review

One a scale of 1 to 5 (low to high), rate the following areas of your performance during this session:

FOCUS: 1 2 3 4 5

EVENNESS OF BREATH: 1 2 3 4 5

BALANCE: 1 2 3 4 5

STRENGTH: 1 2 3 4 5

ENERGY LEVEL: 1 2 3 4 5

ATTITUDE: 1 2 3 4 5

DATE   /   /   TIME   -

☐ **Group Class Practice**

☐ **Home Practice and/or Private Instruction**

NAME OF STUDIO: (OR)   IN WHAT ROOM/SPACE DID YOU PRACTICE?

NAME OF TEACHER:

TEACHER RATING (CIRCLE ONE): A+ A A- B C D F

CLASS LEVEL:
☐ BEGINNER   ☐ INTERMEDIATE   ☐ ADVANCED

CROWD LEVEL: ①②③④⑤
             NOT CROWDED ▸ CROWDED

TEMPERATURE: ☐ HEATED   ☐ UNHEATED

ON WHAT PART OF THE BODY DID YOU FOCUS DURING THIS SESSION?
☐ ABDOMINALS   ☐ HIPS
☐ BACK   ☐ BUTTOCKS
☐ SHOULDERS   ☐ LEGS
☐ ARMS   ☐ ANKLES/FEET
☐ WRISTS/HANDS   ☐ OTHER:

Session Details

WHAT STYLE DID YOU PRACTICE DURING THIS SESSION?
☐ ANUSARA   ☐ KRIPALU
☐ ASHTANGA   ☐ KUNDALINI
☐ BIKRAM   ☐ POWER
☐ IYENGAR   ☐ RESTORATIVE
☐ JIVAMUKTI   ☐ VINIYOGA
                 ☐ OTHER:

WHAT TOOLS DID YOU HAVE ON HAND?
☐ MAT   ☐ STRAP
☐ WATER BOTTLE   ☐ BLANKET
☐ TOWEL   ☐ BOLSTER PILLOW
☐ BLOCK   ☐ OTHER:

SOUND ACCOMPANIMENT: ☐ NO MUSIC   ☐ MUSIC

FAVORITE TRACK FROM TODAY'S SESSION
(TURN TO PAGE 20 AND ADD THE SONG TO YOUR YOGA SOUNDTRACK.)

Overall Session Rating

PACE OF FLOW: ①②③④⑤

DYNAMISM OF SEQUENCING: ①②③④⑤

DIFFICULTY: ①②③④⑤

POSES INCLUDED IN TODAY'S SEQUENCING:
☐ STANDING POSES   ☐ FORWARD BENDS
☐ BALANCING POSES   ☐ BACKBENDS
☐ SEATED POSES   ☐ INVERSIONS
☐ ABDOMINAL STRENGTHENERS   ☐ RESTING POSES
☐ TWISTS

FAVORITE POSE OF TODAY'S SESSION:

MOST CHALLENGING POSE:

POSE YOU HADN'T TRIED BEFORE TODAY:

POSE IN WHICH YOU SHOWED THE MOST IMPROVEMENT:

POSE YOU'D LIKE TO WORK ON IN THE NEXT SESSION:

Dedication

TO WHOM OR WHAT DID YOU DEDICATE THIS CLASS?
(TURN TO PAGE 18 AND ADD YOUR ANSWER TO YOUR DEDICATION LOG.)

Notes and Takeaways

Self-Review

One a scale of 1 to 5 (low to high), rate the following areas of your performance during this session:

FOCUS:	1	2	3	4	5
EVENNESS OF BREATH:	1	2	3	4	5
BALANCE:	1	2	3	4	5
STRENGTH:	1	2	3	4	5
ENERGY LEVEL:	1	2	3	4	5
ATTITUDE:	1	2	3	4	5

DATE   /   /   TIME   -

☐ **Group Class Practice**

☐ **Home Practice and/or Private Instruction**

(OR)

NAME OF STUDIO: IN WHAT ROOM/SPACE DID YOU PRACTICE?

NAME OF TEACHER:

TEACHER RATING (CIRCLE ONE): A+ A A- B C D F

CLASS LEVEL:
☐ BEGINNER   ☐ INTERMEDIATE   ☐ ADVANCED

CROWD LEVEL: 1 2 3 4 5
              NOT CROWDED ► CROWDED

TEMPERATURE: ☐ HEATED   ☐ UNHEATED

ON WHAT PART OF THE BODY DID YOU FOCUS DURING THIS SESSION?

☐ ABDOMINALS   ☐ HIPS
☐ BACK   ☐ BUTTOCKS
☐ SHOULDERS   ☐ LEGS
☐ ARMS   ☐ ANKLES/FEET
☐ WRISTS/HANDS ☐ OTHER:

Session Details

WHAT STYLE DID YOU PRACTICE DURING THIS SESSION?

☐ ANUSARA   ☐ KRIPALU
☐ ASHTANGA   ☐ KUNDALINI
☐ BIKRAM   ☐ POWER
☐ IYENGAR   ☐ RESTORATIVE
☐ JIVAMUKTI   ☐ VINIYOGA
                 ☐ OTHER:

WHAT TOOLS DID YOU HAVE ON HAND?

☐ MAT   ☐ STRAP
☐ WATER BOTTLE   ☐ BLANKET
☐ TOWEL   ☐ BOLSTER PILLOW
☐ BLOCK   ☐ OTHER:

SOUND ACCOMPANIMENT: ☐ NO MUSIC   ☐ MUSIC

FAVORITE TRACK FROM TODAY'S SESSION

Overall Session Rating

PACE OF FLOW: 1 2 3 4 5

DYNAMISM OF SEQUENCING: 1 2 3 4 5

DIFFICULTY: 1 2 3 4 5

POSES INCLUDED IN TODAY'S SEQUENCING:

☐ STANDING POSES   ☐ FORWARD BENDS
☐ BALANCING POSES   ☐ BACKBENDS
☐ SEATED POSES   ☐ INVERSIONS
☐ ABDOMINAL STRENGTHENERS   ☐ RESTING POSES
☐ TWISTS

FAVORITE POSE OF TODAY'S SESSION:

MOST CHALLENGING POSE:

POSE YOU HADN'T TRIED BEFORE TODAY:

POSE IN WHICH YOU SHOWED THE MOST IMPROVEMENT:

POSE YOU'D LIKE TO WORK ON IN THE NEXT SESSION:

Dedication

TO WHOM OR WHAT DID YOU DEDICATE THIS CLASS?
(TURN TO PAGE 18 AND ADD YOUR ANSWER TO YOUR DEDICATION LOG.)

Notes and Takeaways

Self-Review

One a scale of 1 to 5 (low to high), rate the following areas of your performance during this session:

FOCUS: 1 2 3 4 5

EVENNESS
OF BREATH: 1 2 3 4 5

BALANCE: 1 2 3 4 5

STRENGTH: 1 2 3 4 5

ENERGY
LEVEL: 1 2 3 4 5

ATTITUDE: 1 2 3 4 5

Yoga Session 26

DATE   /   /   TIME   -

☐ **Group Class Practice**   ☐ **Home Practice and/or Private Instruction**

NAME OF STUDIO: _____   (OR)   IN WHAT ROOM/SPACE DID YOU PRACTICE?

NAME OF TEACHER: _____

TEACHER RATING (CIRCLE ONE): A+ A A- B C D F   ON WHAT PART OF THE BODY DID YOU FOCUS DURING THIS SESSION?

CLASS LEVEL:
☐ BEGINNER ☐ INTERMEDIATE ☐ ADVANCED   ☐ ABDOMINALS   ☐ HIPS
                                             ☐ BACK   ☐ BUTTOCKS
CROWD LEVEL: ①②③④⑤   ☐ SHOULDERS   ☐ LEGS
           NOT CROWDED ▸ CROWDED   ☐ ARMS   ☐ ANKLES/FEET
TEMPERATURE: ☐ HEATED ☐ UNHEATED   ☐ WRISTS/HANDS   ☐ OTHER: _____

Session Details

WHAT STYLE DID YOU PRACTICE DURING THIS SESSION?   WHAT TOOLS DID YOU HAVE ON HAND?

☐ ANUSARA   ☐ KRIPALU   ☐ MAT   ☐ STRAP
☐ ASHTANGA   ☐ KUNDALINI   ☐ WATER BOTTLE   ☐ BLANKET
☐ BIKRAM   ☐ POWER   ☐ TOWEL   ☐ BOLSTER PILLOW
☐ IYENGAR   ☐ RESTORATIVE   ☐ BLOCK   ☐ OTHER: _____
☐ JIVAMUKTI   ☐ VINIYOGA
                ☐ OTHER: _____

SOUND ACCOMPANIMENT: ☐ NO MUSIC ☐ MUSIC

FAVORITE TRACK FROM TODAY'S SESSION
(TURN TO PAGE 20 AND ADD THE SONG TO YOUR YOGA SOUNDTRACK.)

Overall Session Rating

PACE OF FLOW: ①②③④⑤   FAVORITE POSE OF TODAY'S SESSION:

DYNAMISM OF SEQUENCING: ①②③④⑤
                                          MOST CHALLENGING POSE:
DIFFICULTY: ①②③④⑤

POSES INCLUDED IN TODAY'S SEQUENCING: POSE YOU HADN'T TRIED BEFORE TODAY:

☐ STANDING POSES   ☐ FORWARD BENDS
☐ BALANCING POSES   ☐ BACKBENDS   POSE IN WHICH YOU SHOWED THE MOST IMPROVEMENT:
☐ SEATED POSES   ☐ INVERSIONS
☐ ABDOMINAL   ☐ RESTING POSES
  STRENGTHENERS   POSE YOU'D LIKE TO WORK ON IN THE NEXT SESSION:
☐ TWISTS

Dedication

TO WHOM OR WHAT DID YOU DEDICATE THIS CLASS?
(TURN TO PAGE 18 AND ADD YOUR ANSWER TO YOUR DEDICATION LOG.)

Notes and Takeaways

Self-Review

One a scale of 1 to 5 (low to high), rate the following areas of your performance during this session:

FOCUS:	1	2	3	4	5
EVENNESS OF BREATH:	1	2	3	4	5
BALANCE:	1	2	3	4	5
STRENGTH:	1	2	3	4	5
ENERGY LEVEL:	1	2	3	4	5
ATTITUDE:	1	2	3	4	5

Yoga Session 27

DATE   /   /   TIME   -

☐ **Group Class Practice**

NAME OF STUDIO:

NAME OF TEACHER:

TEACHER RATING (CIRCLE ONE): A+ A A- B C D F

CLASS LEVEL:
☐ BEGINNER ☐ INTERMEDIATE ☐ ADVANCED

CROWD LEVEL: 1 2 3 4 5
          NOT CROWDED ▸ CROWDED

TEMPERATURE: ☐ HEATED ☐ UNHEATED

(OR)

☐ **Home Practice and/or Private Instruction**

IN WHAT ROOM/SPACE DID YOU PRACTICE?

ON WHAT PART OF THE BODY DID YOU FOCUS DURING THIS SESSION?

☐ ABDOMINALS   ☐ HIPS
☐ BACK   ☐ BUTTOCKS
☐ SHOULDERS   ☐ LEGS
☐ ARMS   ☐ ANKLES/FEET
☐ WRISTS/HANDS   ☐ OTHER:

Session Details

WHAT STYLE DID YOU PRACTICE DURING THIS SESSION?

☐ ANUSARA   ☐ KRIPALU
☐ ASHTANGA   ☐ KUNDALINI
☐ BIKRAM   ☐ POWER
☐ IYENGAR   ☐ RESTORATIVE
☐ JIVAMUKTI   ☐ VINIYOGA
               ☐ OTHER:

WHAT TOOLS DID YOU HAVE ON HAND?

☐ MAT   ☐ STRAP
☐ WATER BOTTLE   ☐ BLANKET
☐ TOWEL   ☐ BOLSTER PILLOW
☐ BLOCK   ☐ OTHER:

SOUND ACCOMPANIMENT: ☐ NO MUSIC ☐ MUSIC

FAVORITE TRACK FROM TODAY'S SESSION
(TURN TO PAGE 20 AND ADD THE SONG TO YOUR YOGA SOUNDTRACK.)

Overall Session Rating

PACE OF FLOW: 1 2 3 4 5

DYNAMISM OF SEQUENCING: 1 2 3 4 5

DIFFICULTY: 1 2 3 4 5

POSES INCLUDED IN TODAY'S SEQUENCING:

☐ STANDING POSES   ☐ FORWARD BENDS
☐ BALANCING POSES   ☐ BACKBENDS
☐ SEATED POSES   ☐ INVERSIONS
☐ ABDOMINAL STRENGTHENERS ☐ RESTING POSES
☐ TWISTS

FAVORITE POSE OF TODAY'S SESSION:

MOST CHALLENGING POSE:

POSE YOU HADN'T TRIED BEFORE TODAY:

POSE IN WHICH YOU SHOWED THE MOST IMPROVEMENT:

POSE YOU'D LIKE TO WORK ON IN THE NEXT SESSION:

Dedication

TO WHOM OR WHAT DID YOU DEDICATE THIS CLASS?
(TURN TO PAGE 18 AND ADD YOUR ANSWER TO YOUR DEDICATION LOG.)

Notes and Takeaways

Self-Review

One a scale of 1 to 5 (low to high), rate the following areas of your performance during this session:

FOCUS: 1 2 3 4 5

EVENNESS
OF BREATH: 1 2 3 4 5

BALANCE: 1 2 3 4 5

STRENGTH: 1 2 3 4 5

ENERGY
LEVEL: 1 2 3 4 5

ATTITUDE: 1 2 3 4 5

DATE   /   /   TIME   -

☐ **Group Class Practice**

NAME OF STUDIO:

NAME OF TEACHER:

TEACHER RATING (CIRCLE ONE): A+ A A- B C D F

CLASS LEVEL:
☐ BEGINNER   ☐ INTERMEDIATE   ☐ ADVANCED

CROWD LEVEL: 1 2 3 4 5
                   NOT CROWDED ▶ CROWDED

TEMPERATURE: ☐ HEATED   ☐ UNHEATED

☐ **Home Practice and/or Private Instruction**

(OR)   IN WHAT ROOM/SPACE DID YOU PRACTICE?

ON WHAT PART OF THE BODY DID YOU FOCUS DURING THIS SESSION?

☐ ABDOMINALS   ☐ HIPS
☐ BACK   ☐ BUTTOCKS
☐ SHOULDERS   ☐ LEGS
☐ ARMS   ☐ ANKLES/FEET
☐ WRISTS/HANDS ☐ OTHER:

Session Details

WHAT STYLE DID YOU PRACTICE DURING THIS SESSION?

☐ ANUSARA   ☐ KRIPALU
☐ ASHTANGA   ☐ KUNDALINI
☐ BIKRAM   ☐ POWER
☐ IYENGAR   ☐ RESTORATIVE
☐ JIVAMUKTI   ☐ VINIYOGA
                ☐ OTHER:

SOUND ACCOMPANIMENT: ☐ NO MUSIC   ☐ MUSIC

FAVORITE TRACK FROM TODAY'S SESSION
(TURN TO PAGE 28 AND ADD THE SONG TO YOUR YOGA SOUNDTRACK.)

WHAT TOOLS DID YOU HAVE ON HAND?

☐ MAT   ☐ STRAP
☐ WATER BOTTLE   ☐ BLANKET
☐ TOWEL   ☐ BOLSTER PILLOW
☐ BLOCK   ☐ OTHER:

Overall Session Rating

PACE OF FLOW: 1 2 3 4 5

DYNAMISM OF SEQUENCING: 1 2 3 4 5

DIFFICULTY: 1 2 3 4 5

POSES INCLUDED IN TODAY'S SEQUENCING:

☐ STANDING POSES   ☐ FORWARD BENDS
☐ BALANCING POSES   ☐ BACKBENDS
☐ SEATED POSES   ☐ INVERSIONS
☐ ABDOMINAL STRENGTHENERS   ☐ RESTING POSES
☐ TWISTS

FAVORITE POSE OF TODAY'S SESSION:

MOST CHALLENGING POSE:

POSE YOU HADN'T TRIED BEFORE TODAY:

POSE IN WHICH YOU SHOWED THE MOST IMPROVEMENT:

POSE YOU'D LIKE TO WORK ON IN THE NEXT SESSION:

Dedication

TO WHOM OR WHAT DID YOU DEDICATE THIS CLASS?
(TURN TO PAGE 18 AND ADD YOUR ANSWER TO YOUR DEDICATION LOG.)

Notes and Takeaways

Self-Review

One a scale of 1 to 5 (low to high), rate the following areas of your performance during this session:

FOCUS: 1 2 3 4 5

EVENNESS
OF BREATH: 1 2 3 4 5

BALANCE: 1 2 3 4 5

STRENGTH: 1 2 3 4 5

ENERGY
LEVEL: 1 2 3 4 5

ATTITUDE: 1 2 3 4 5

DATE   /   /   TIME   -

☐ **Group Class Practice**

☐ **Home Practice and/or Private Instruction**

(OR)

NAME OF STUDIO:

IN WHAT ROOM/SPACE DID YOU PRACTICE?

NAME OF TEACHER:

TEACHER RATING (CIRCLE ONE): A+ A A- B C D F

CLASS LEVEL:

☐ BEGINNER ☐ INTERMEDIATE ☐ ADVANCED

CROWD LEVEL: 1 2 3 4 5
                NOT CROWDED ▸ CROWDED

TEMPERATURE: ☐ HEATED ☐ UNHEATED

ON WHAT PART OF THE BODY DID YOU FOCUS DURING THIS SESSION?

☐ ABDOMINALS   ☐ HIPS
☐ BACK   ☐ BUTTOCKS
☐ SHOULDERS   ☐ LEGS
☐ ARMS   ☐ ANKLES/FEET
☐ WRISTS/HANDS ☐ OTHER:

Session Details

WHAT STYLE DID YOU PRACTICE DURING THIS SESSION?

☐ ANUSARA   ☐ KRIPALU
☐ ASHTANGA   ☐ KUNDALINI
☐ BIKRAM   ☐ POWER
☐ IYENGAR   ☐ RESTORATIVE
☐ JIVAMUKTI   ☐ VINIYOGA
               ☐ OTHER:

WHAT TOOLS DID YOU HAVE ON HAND?

☐ MAT   ☐ STRAP
☐ WATER BOTTLE   ☐ BLANKET
☐ TOWEL   ☐ BOLSTER PILLOW
☐ BLOCK   ☐ OTHER:

SOUND ACCOMPANIMENT: ☐ NO MUSIC ☐ MUSIC

FAVORITE TRACK FROM TODAY'S SESSION
(TURN TO PAGE 20 AND ADD THE SONG TO YOUR YOGA SOUNDTRACK.)

Overall Session Rating

PACE OF FLOW: 1 2 3 4 5

DYNAMISM OF SEQUENCING: 1 2 3 4 5

DIFFICULTY: 1 2 3 4 5

POSES INCLUDED IN TODAY'S SEQUENCING:

☐ STANDING POSES   ☐ FORWARD BENDS
☐ BALANCING POSES   ☐ BACKBENDS
☐ SEATED POSES   ☐ INVERSIONS
☐ ABDOMINAL STRENGTHENERS ☐ RESTING POSES
☐ TWISTS

FAVORITE POSE OF TODAY'S SESSION:

MOST CHALLENGING POSE:

POSE YOU HADN'T TRIED BEFORE TODAY:

POSE IN WHICH YOU SHOWED THE MOST IMPROVEMENT:

POSE YOU'D LIKE TO WORK ON IN THE NEXT SESSION:

Dedication

TO WHOM OR WHAT DID YOU DEDICATE THIS CLASS?
(TURN TO PAGE 18 AND ADD YOUR ANSWER TO YOUR DEDICATION LOG.)

Notes and Takeaways

Self-Review

One a scale of 1 to 5 (low to high), rate the following areas of your performance during this session:

FOCUS: 1 2 3 4 5

EVENNESS OF BREATH: 1 2 3 4 5

BALANCE: 1 2 3 4 5

STRENGTH: 1 2 3 4 5

ENERGY LEVEL: 1 2 3 4 5

ATTITUDE: 1 2 3 4 5

DATE   /   /   TIME   -

☐ **Group Class Practice**

☐ **Home Practice and/or Private Instruction**

(OR)

NAME OF STUDIO: IN WHAT ROOM/SPACE DID YOU PRACTICE?

NAME OF TEACHER:

TEACHER RATING (CIRCLE ONE): A+ A A- B C D F

CLASS LEVEL:
☐ BEGINNER ☐ INTERMEDIATE ☐ ADVANCED

CROWD LEVEL: 1 2 3 4 5
            NOT CROWDED → CROWDED

TEMPERATURE: ☐ HEATED ☐ UNHEATED

ON WHAT PART OF THE BODY DID YOU FOCUS DURING THIS SESSION?
☐ ABDOMINALS   ☐ HIPS
☐ BACK   ☐ BUTTOCKS
☐ SHOULDERS   ☐ LEGS
☐ ARMS   ☐ ANKLES/FEET
☐ WRISTS/HANDS   ☐ OTHER:

Session Details

WHAT STYLE DID YOU PRACTICE DURING THIS SESSION?
☐ ANUSARA   ☐ KRIPALU
☐ ASHTANGA   ☐ KUNDALINI
☐ BIKRAM   ☐ POWER
☐ IYENGAR   ☐ RESTORATIVE
☐ JIVAMUKTI   ☐ VINIYOGA
                ☐ OTHER:

WHAT TOOLS DID YOU HAVE ON HAND?
☐ MAT   ☐ STRAP
☐ WATER BOTTLE   ☐ BLANKET
☐ TOWEL   ☐ BOLSTER PILLOW
☐ BLOCK   ☐ OTHER:

SOUND ACCOMPANIMENT: ☐ NO MUSIC ☐ MUSIC

FAVORITE TRACK FROM TODAY'S SESSION
(TURN TO PAGE 20 AND ADD THE SONG TO YOUR YOGA SOUNDTRACK.)

Overall Session Rating

PACE OF FLOW: 1 2 3 4 5

DYNAMISM OF SEQUENCING: 1 2 3 4 5

DIFFICULTY: 1 2 3 4 5

POSES INCLUDED IN TODAY'S SEQUENCING:
☐ STANDING POSES   ☐ FORWARD BENDS
☐ BALANCING POSES   ☐ BACKBENDS
☐ SEATED POSES   ☐ INVERSIONS
☐ ABDOMINAL STRENGTHENERS ☐ RESTING POSES
☐ TWISTS

FAVORITE POSE OF TODAY'S SESSION:

MOST CHALLENGING POSE:

POSE YOU HADN'T TRIED BEFORE TODAY:

POSE IN WHICH YOU SHOWED THE MOST IMPROVEMENT:

POSE YOU'D LIKE TO WORK ON IN THE NEXT SESSION:

Dedication

TO WHOM OR WHAT DID YOU DEDICATE THIS CLASS?
(TURN TO PAGE 18 AND ADD YOUR ANSWER TO YOUR DEDICATION LOG.)

Notes and Takeaways

Self-Review

One a scale of 1 to 5 (low to high), rate the following areas of your performance during this session:

FOCUS: 1 2 3 4 5

EVENNESS
OF BREATH: 1 2 3 4 5

BALANCE: 1 2 3 4 5

STRENGTH: 1 2 3 4 5

ENERGY
LEVEL: 1 2 3 4 5

ATTITUDE: 1 2 3 4 5

DATE   /   /   TIME   -

☐ **Group Class Practice**

☐ **Home Practice and/or Private Instruction**

NAME OF STUDIO:

(OR) IN WHAT ROOM/SPACE DID YOU PRACTICE?

NAME OF TEACHER:

TEACHER RATING (CIRCLE ONE): A+ A A- B C D F

CLASS LEVEL:
☐ BEGINNER ☐ INTERMEDIATE ☐ ADVANCED

CROWD LEVEL: (1) (2) (3) (4) (5)
          NOT CROWDED ▸ CROWDED

TEMPERATURE: ☐ HEATED ☐ UNHEATED

ON WHAT PART OF THE BODY DID YOU FOCUS DURING THIS SESSION?

☐ ABDOMINALS   ☐ HIPS
☐ BACK   ☐ BUTTOCKS
☐ SHOULDERS   ☐ LEGS
☐ ARMS   ☐ ANKLES/FEET
☐ WRISTS/HANDS ☐ OTHER:

Session Details

WHAT STYLE DID YOU PRACTICE DURING THIS SESSION?

☐ ANUSARA   ☐ KRIPALU
☐ ASHTANGA   ☐ KUNDALINI
☐ BIKRAM   ☐ POWER
☐ IYENGAR   ☐ RESTORATIVE
☐ JIVAMUKTI   ☐ VINIYOGA
               ☐ OTHER:

WHAT TOOLS DID YOU HAVE ON HAND?

☐ MAT   ☐ STRAP
☐ WATER BOTTLE ☐ BLANKET
☐ TOWEL   ☐ BOLSTER PILLOW
☐ BLOCK   ☐ OTHER:

SOUND ACCOMPANIMENT: ☐ NO MUSIC ☐ MUSIC

FAVORITE TRACK FROM TODAY'S SESSION
(TURN TO PAGE 20 AND ADD THE SONG TO YOUR YOGA SOUNDTRACK.)

Overall Session Rating

PACE OF FLOW: (1) (2) (3) (4) (5)

DYNAMISM OF SEQUENCING: (1) (2) (3) (4) (5)

DIFFICULTY: (1) (2) (3) (4) (5)

POSES INCLUDED IN TODAY'S SEQUENCING:

☐ STANDING POSES   ☐ FORWARD BENDS
☐ BALANCING POSES   ☐ BACKBENDS
☐ SEATED POSES   ☐ INVERSIONS
☐ ABDOMINAL STRENGTHENERS ☐ RESTING POSES
☐ TWISTS

FAVORITE POSE OF TODAY'S SESSION:

MOST CHALLENGING POSE:

POSE YOU HADN'T TRIED BEFORE TODAY:

POSE IN WHICH YOU SHOWED THE MOST IMPROVEMENT:

POSE YOU'D LIKE TO WORK ON IN THE NEXT SESSION:

Dedication

TO WHOM OR WHAT DID YOU DEDICATE THIS CLASS?
(TURN TO PAGE 18 AND ADD YOUR ANSWER TO YOUR DEDICATION LOG.)

Notes and Takeaways

Self-Review

One a scale of 1 to 5 (low to high), rate the following areas of your performance during this session:

FOCUS: 1 2 3 4 5

EVENNESS
OF BREATH: 1 2 3 4 5

BALANCE: 1 2 3 4 5

STRENGTH: 1 2 3 4 5

ENERGY
LEVEL: 1 2 3 4 5

ATTITUDE: 1 2 3 4 5

DATE   /   /   TIME   -

☐ **Group Class Practice**

☐ **Home Practice and/or Private Instruction**

(OR)

NAME OF STUDIO:

IN WHAT ROOM/SPACE DID YOU PRACTICE?

NAME OF TEACHER:

TEACHER RATING (CIRCLE ONE): A+ A A- B C D F

CLASS LEVEL:
☐ BEGINNER   ☐ INTERMEDIATE   ☐ ADVANCED

CROWD LEVEL: 1   2   3   4   5
        NOT CROWDED → CROWDED

TEMPERATURE: ☐ HEATED   ☐ UNHEATED

ON WHAT PART OF THE BODY DID YOU FOCUS DURING THIS SESSION?

☐ ABDOMINALS   ☐ HIPS
☐ BACK   ☐ BUTTOCKS
☐ SHOULDERS   ☐ LEGS
☐ ARMS   ☐ ANKLES/FEET
☐ WRISTS/HANDS   ☐ OTHER:

Session Details

WHAT STYLE DID YOU PRACTICE DURING THIS SESSION?

☐ ANUSARA   ☐ KRIPALU
☐ ASHTANGA   ☐ KUNDALINI
☐ BIKRAM   ☐ POWER
☐ IYENGAR   ☐ RESTORATIVE
☐ JIVAMUKTI   ☐ VINIYOGA
            ☐ OTHER:

WHAT TOOLS DID YOU HAVE ON HAND?

☐ MAT   ☐ STRAP
☐ WATER BOTTLE   ☐ BLANKET
☐ TOWEL   ☐ BOLSTER PILLOW
☐ BLOCK   ☐ OTHER:

SOUND ACCOMPANIMENT: ☐ NO MUSIC   ☐ MUSIC

FAVORITE TRACK FROM TODAY'S SESSION
(TURN TO PAGE 20 AND ADD THE SONG TO YOUR YOGA SOUNDTRACK.)

Overall Session Rating

PACE OF FLOW: 1   2   3   4   5

DYNAMISM OF SEQUENCING: 1   2   3   4   5

DIFFICULTY: 1   2   3   4   5

POSES INCLUDED IN TODAY'S SEQUENCING:

☐ STANDING POSES   ☐ FORWARD BENDS
☐ BALANCING POSES   ☐ BACKBENDS
☐ SEATED POSES   ☐ INVERSIONS
☐ ABDOMINAL STRENGTHENERS   ☐ RESTING POSES
☐ TWISTS

FAVORITE POSE OF TODAY'S SESSION:

MOST CHALLENGING POSE:

POSE YOU HADN'T TRIED BEFORE TODAY:

POSE IN WHICH YOU SHOWED THE MOST IMPROVEMENT:

POSE YOU'D LIKE TO WORK ON IN THE NEXT SESSION:

Dedication

TO WHOM OR WHAT DID YOU DEDICATE THIS CLASS?
(TURN TO PAGE 18 AND ADD YOUR ANSWER TO YOUR DEDICATION LOG.)

Notes and Takeaways

Self-Review

One a scale of 1 to 5 (low to high), rate the following areas of your performance during this session:

FOCUS:	1	2	3	4	5
EVENNESS OF BREATH:	1	2	3	4	5
BALANCE:	1	2	3	4	5
STRENGTH:	1	2	3	4	5
ENERGY LEVEL:	1	2	3	4	5
ATTITUDE:	1	2	3	4	5

Yoga Session 33

DATE / / TIME -

☐ **Group Class Practice**

☐ **Home Practice and/or Private Instruction**

(OR)

NAME OF STUDIO:

IN WHAT ROOM/SPACE DID YOU PRACTICE?

NAME OF TEACHER:

TEACHER RATING (CIRCLE ONE): A+ A A- B C D F

ON WHAT PART OF THE BODY DID YOU FOCUS DURING THIS SESSION?

CLASS LEVEL:
☐ BEGINNER ☐ INTERMEDIATE ☐ ADVANCED

☐ ABDOMINALS ☐ HIPS
☐ BACK ☐ BUTTOCKS

CROWD LEVEL: 1 2 3 4 5
NOT CROWDED ▸ CROWDED

☐ SHOULDERS ☐ LEGS
☐ ARMS ☐ ANKLES/FEET

TEMPERATURE: ☐ HEATED ☐ UNHEATED

☐ WRISTS/HANDS ☐ OTHER:

Session Details

WHAT STYLE DID YOU PRACTICE DURING THIS SESSION?

☐ ANUSARA ☐ KRIPALU
☐ ASHTANGA ☐ KUNDALINI
☐ BIKRAM ☐ POWER
☐ IYENGAR ☐ RESTORATIVE
☐ JIVAMUKTI ☐ VINIYOGA
☐ OTHER:

WHAT TOOLS DID YOU HAVE ON HAND?

☐ MAT ☐ STRAP
☐ WATER BOTTLE ☐ BLANKET
☐ TOWEL ☐ BOLSTER PILLOW
☐ BLOCK ☐ OTHER:

SOUND ACCOMPANIMENT: ☐ NO MUSIC ☐ MUSIC

FAVORITE TRACK FROM TODAY'S SESSION
(TURN TO PAGE 20 AND ADD THE SONG TO YOUR YOGA SOUNDTRACK.)

Overall Session Rating

PACE OF FLOW: 1 2 3 4 5

FAVORITE POSE OF TODAY'S SESSION:

DYNAMISM OF SEQUENCING: 1 2 3 4 5

MOST CHALLENGING POSE:

DIFFICULTY: 1 2 3 4 5

POSE YOU HADN'T TRIED BEFORE TODAY:

POSES INCLUDED IN TODAY'S SEQUENCING:
☐ STANDING POSES ☐ FORWARD BENDS
☐ BALANCING POSES ☐ BACKBENDS
☐ SEATED POSES ☐ INVERSIONS
☐ ABDOMINAL STRENGTHENERS ☐ RESTING POSES
☐ TWISTS

POSE IN WHICH YOU SHOWED THE MOST IMPROVEMENT:

POSE YOU'D LIKE TO WORK ON IN THE NEXT SESSION:

Dedication

TO WHOM OR WHAT DID YOU DEDICATE THIS CLASS?
(TURN TO PAGE 18 AND ADD YOUR ANSWER TO YOUR DEDICATION LOG.)

Notes and Takeaways

Self-Review

One a scale of 1 to 5 (low to high), rate the following areas of your performance during this session:

FOCUS: 1 2 3 4 5

EVENNESS
OF BREATH: 1 2 3 4 5

BALANCE: 1 2 3 4 5

STRENGTH: 1 2 3 4 5

ENERGY
LEVEL: 1 2 3 4 5

ATTITUDE: 1 2 3 4 5

Yoga Session (34)

DATE   /   /   TIME   -

☐ **Group Class Practice**

NAME OF STUDIO:

NAME OF TEACHER:

TEACHER RATING (CIRCLE ONE): A+ A A- B C D F

CLASS LEVEL:
☐ BEGINNER   ☐ INTERMEDIATE   ☐ ADVANCED

CROWD LEVEL: 1 2 3 4 5
            NOT CROWDED → CROWDED

TEMPERATURE: ☐ HEATED   ☐ UNHEATED

OR

☐ **Home Practice and/or Private Instruction**

IN WHAT ROOM/SPACE DID YOU PRACTICE?

ON WHAT PART OF THE BODY DID YOU FOCUS DURING THIS SESSION?

☐ ABDOMINALS   ☐ HIPS
☐ BACK   ☐ BUTTOCKS
☐ SHOULDERS   ☐ LEGS
☐ ARMS   ☐ ANKLES/FEET
☐ WRISTS/HANDS   ☐ OTHER:

Session Details

WHAT STYLE DID YOU PRACTICE DURING THIS SESSION?

☐ ANUSARA   ☐ KRIPALU
☐ ASHTANGA   ☐ KUNDALINI
☐ BIKRAM   ☐ POWER
☐ IYENGAR   ☐ RESTORATIVE
☐ JIVAMUKTI   ☐ VINIYOGA
               ☐ OTHER:

WHAT TOOLS DID YOU HAVE ON HAND?

☐ MAT   ☐ STRAP
☐ WATER BOTTLE   ☐ BLANKET
☐ TOWEL   ☐ BOLSTER PILLOW
☐ BLOCK   ☐ OTHER:

SOUND ACCOMPANIMENT: ☐ NO MUSIC   ☐ MUSIC

FAVORITE TRACK FROM TODAY'S SESSION
(TURN TO PAGE 28 AND ADD THE SONG TO YOUR YOGA SOUNDTRACK.)

Overall Session Rating

PACE OF FLOW: 1 2 3 4 5

DYNAMISM OF SEQUENCING: 1 2 3 4 5

DIFFICULTY: 1 2 3 4 5

POSES INCLUDED IN TODAY'S SEQUENCING:

☐ STANDING POSES   ☐ FORWARD BENDS
☐ BALANCING POSES   ☐ BACKBENDS
☐ SEATED POSES   ☐ INVERSIONS
☐ ABDOMINAL STRENGTHENERS ☐ RESTING POSES
☐ TWISTS

FAVORITE POSE OF TODAY'S SESSION:

MOST CHALLENGING POSE:

POSE YOU HADN'T TRIED BEFORE TODAY:

POSE IN WHICH YOU SHOWED THE MOST IMPROVEMENT:

POSE YOU'D LIKE TO WORK ON IN THE NEXT SESSION:

Dedication

TO WHOM OR WHAT DID YOU DEDICATE THIS CLASS?
(TURN TO PAGE 18 AND ADD YOUR ANSWER TO YOUR DEDICATION LOG.)

Notes and Takeaways

Self-Review

One a scale of 1 to 5 (low to high), rate the following areas of your performance during this session:

FOCUS:	1	2	3	4	5
EVENNESS OF BREATH:	1	2	3	4	5
BALANCE:	1	2	3	4	5
STRENGTH:	1	2	3	4	5
ENERGY LEVEL:	1	2	3	4	5
ATTITUDE:	1	2	3	4	5

DATE   /   /   TIME   -

☐ **Group Class Practice**

☐ **Home Practice and/or Private Instruction**

NAME OF STUDIO:

NAME OF TEACHER:

(OR) **IN WHAT ROOM/SPACE DID YOU PRACTICE?**

TEACHER RATING (CIRCLE ONE): A+ A A- B C D F

CLASS LEVEL:

☐ BEGINNER ☐ INTERMEDIATE ☐ ADVANCED

CROWD LEVEL: 1 2 3 4 5
          NOT CROWDED ▸ CROWDED

TEMPERATURE: ☐ HEATED ☐ UNHEATED

ON WHAT PART OF THE BODY DID YOU FOCUS DURING THIS SESSION?

☐ ABDOMINALS   ☐ HIPS
☐ BACK   ☐ BUTTOCKS
☐ SHOULDERS   ☐ LEGS
☐ ARMS   ☐ ANKLES/FEET
☐ WRISTS/HANDS ☐ OTHER:

Session Details

WHAT STYLE DID YOU PRACTICE DURING THIS SESSION?

☐ ANUSARA   ☐ KRIPALU
☐ ASHTANGA   ☐ KUNDALINI
☐ BIKRAM   ☐ POWER
☐ IYENGAR   ☐ RESTORATIVE
☐ JIVAMUKTI   ☐ VINIYOGA
              ☐ OTHER:

WHAT TOOLS DID YOU HAVE ON HAND?

☐ MAT   ☐ STRAP
☐ WATER BOTTLE   ☐ BLANKET
☐ TOWEL   ☐ BOLSTER PILLOW
☐ BLOCK   ☐ OTHER:

SOUND ACCOMPANIMENT: ☐ NO MUSIC ☐ MUSIC

FAVORITE TRACK FROM TODAY'S SESSION
(TURN TO PAGE 20 AND ADD THE SONG TO YOUR YOGA SOUNDTRACK.)

Overall Session Rating

PACE OF FLOW: 1 2 3 4 5

DYNAMISM OF SEQUENCING: 1 2 3 4 5

DIFFICULTY: 1 2 3 4 5

POSES INCLUDED IN TODAY'S SEQUENCING:

☐ STANDING POSES   ☐ FORWARD BENDS
☐ BALANCING POSES   ☐ BACKBENDS
☐ SEATED POSES   ☐ INVERSIONS
☐ ABDOMINAL STRENGTHENERS ☐ RESTING POSES
☐ TWISTS

FAVORITE POSE OF TODAY'S SESSION:

MOST CHALLENGING POSE:

POSE YOU HADN'T TRIED BEFORE TODAY:

POSE IN WHICH YOU SHOWED THE MOST IMPROVEMENT:

POSE YOU'D LIKE TO WORK ON IN THE NEXT SESSION:

Dedication

TO WHOM OR WHAT DID YOU DEDICATE THIS CLASS?
(TURN TO PAGE 18 AND ADD YOUR ANSWER TO YOUR DEDICATION LOG.)

Notes and Takeaways

Self-Review

One a scale of 1 to 5 (low to high), rate the following areas of your performance during this session:

FOCUS: 1 2 3 4 5

EVENNESS
OF BREATH: 1 2 3 4 5

BALANCE: 1 2 3 4 5

STRENGTH: 1 2 3 4 5

ENERGY
LEVEL: 1 2 3 4 5

ATTITUDE: 1 2 3 4 5

Yoga Session (36)

DATE   /   /   TIME   -

☐ **Group Class Practice**

NAME OF STUDIO:

NAME OF TEACHER:

TEACHER RATING (CIRCLE ONE): A+ A A- B C D F

CLASS LEVEL:

☐ BEGINNER   ☐ INTERMEDIATE   ☐ ADVANCED

CROWD LEVEL: 1 · 2 · 3 · 4 · 5

　　　　　　NOT CROWDED ▸ CROWDED

TEMPERATURE: ☐ HEATED   ☐ UNHEATED

OR

☐ **Home Practice and/or Private Instruction**

IN WHAT ROOM/SPACE DID YOU PRACTICE?

ON WHAT PART OF THE BODY DID YOU FOCUS DURING THIS SESSION?

☐ ABDOMINALS   ☐ HIPS
☐ BACK   ☐ BUTTOCKS
☐ SHOULDERS   ☐ LEGS
☐ ARMS   ☐ ANKLES/FEET
☐ WRISTS/HANDS   ☐ OTHER:

Session Details

WHAT STYLE DID YOU PRACTICE DURING THIS SESSION?

☐ ANUSARA   ☐ KRIPALU
☐ ASHTANGA   ☐ KUNDALINI
☐ BIKRAM   ☐ POWER
☐ IYENGAR   ☐ RESTORATIVE
☐ JIVAMUKTI   ☐ VINIYOGA
                ☐ OTHER:

SOUND ACCOMPANIMENT: ☐ NO MUSIC   ☐ MUSIC

FAVORITE TRACK FROM TODAY'S SESSION
(TURN TO PAGE 20 AND ADD THE SONG TO YOUR YOGA SOUNDTRACK.)

WHAT TOOLS DID YOU HAVE ON HAND?

☐ MAT   ☐ STRAP
☐ WATER BOTTLE   ☐ BLANKET
☐ TOWEL   ☐ BOLSTER PILLOW
☐ BLOCK   ☐ OTHER:

Overall Session Rating

PACE OF FLOW: 1 · 2 · 3 · 4 · 5

DYNAMISM OF SEQUENCING: 1 · 2 · 3 · 4 · 5

DIFFICULTY: 1 · 2 · 3 · 4 · 5

POSES INCLUDED IN TODAY'S SEQUENCING:

☐ STANDING POSES   ☐ FORWARD BENDS
☐ BALANCING POSES   ☐ BACKBENDS
☐ SEATED POSES   ☐ INVERSIONS
☐ ABDOMINAL STRENGTHENERS   ☐ RESTING POSES
☐ TWISTS

FAVORITE POSE OF TODAY'S SESSION:

MOST CHALLENGING POSE:

POSE YOU HADN'T TRIED BEFORE TODAY:

POSE IN WHICH YOU SHOWED THE MOST IMPROVEMENT:

POSE YOU'D LIKE TO WORK ON IN THE NEXT SESSION:

Dedication

TO WHOM OR WHAT DID YOU DEDICATE THIS CLASS?
(TURN TO PAGE 18 AND ADD YOUR ANSWER TO YOUR DEDICATION LOG.)

Notes and Takeaways

Self-Review

One a scale of 1 to 5 (low to high), rate the following areas of your performance during this session:

FOCUS: 1 2 3 4 5

EVENNESS
OF BREATH: 1 2 3 4 5

BALANCE: 1 2 3 4 5

STRENGTH: 1 2 3 4 5

ENERGY
LEVEL: 1 2 3 4 5

ATTITUDE: 1 2 3 4 5

DATE   /   /   TIME   -

☐ **Group Class Practice**   ☐ **Home Practice and/or Private Instruction**

(OR)

NAME OF STUDIO: IN WHAT ROOM/SPACE DID YOU PRACTICE?

NAME OF TEACHER:

TEACHER RATING (CIRCLE ONE): A+ A A- B C D F   ON WHAT PART OF THE BODY DID YOU FOCUS DURING THIS SESSION?

CLASS LEVEL:
☐ BEGINNER ☐ INTERMEDIATE ☐ ADVANCED

CROWD LEVEL: 1 2 3 4 5

NOT CROWDED ▶ CROWDED

TEMPERATURE: ☐ HEATED ☐ UNHEATED

☐ ABDOMINALS   ☐ HIPS
☐ BACK   ☐ BUTTOCKS
☐ SHOULDERS   ☐ LEGS
☐ ARMS   ☐ ANKLES/FEET
☐ WRISTS/HANDS ☐ OTHER:

Session Details

WHAT STYLE DID YOU PRACTICE DURING THIS SESSION?

☐ ANUSARA   ☐ KRIPALU
☐ ASHTANGA   ☐ KUNDALINI
☐ BIKRAM   ☐ POWER
☐ IYENGAR   ☐ RESTORATIVE
☐ JIVAMUKTI   ☐ VINIYOGA
               ☐ OTHER:

WHAT TOOLS DID YOU HAVE ON HAND?

☐ MAT   ☐ STRAP
☐ WATER BOTTLE ☐ BLANKET
☐ TOWEL   ☐ BOLSTER PILLOW
☐ BLOCK   ☐ OTHER:

SOUND ACCOMPANIMENT: ☐ NO MUSIC   ☐ MUSIC

FAVORITE TRACK FROM TODAY'S SESSION
(TURN TO PAGE 20 AND ADD THE SONG TO YOUR YOGA SOUNDTRACK.)

Overall Session Rating

PACE OF FLOW: 1 2 3 4 5

DYNAMISM OF SEQUENCING: 1 2 3 4 5

DIFFICULTY: 1 2 3 4 5

POSES INCLUDED IN TODAY'S SEQUENCING:

☐ STANDING POSES   ☐ FORWARD BENDS
☐ BALANCING POSES   ☐ BACKBENDS
☐ SEATED POSES   ☐ INVERSIONS
☐ ABDOMINAL STRENGTHENERS ☐ RESTING POSES
☐ TWISTS

FAVORITE POSE OF TODAY'S SESSION:

MOST CHALLENGING POSE:

POSE YOU HADN'T TRIED BEFORE TODAY:

POSE IN WHICH YOU SHOWED THE MOST IMPROVEMENT:

POSE YOU'D LIKE TO WORK ON IN THE NEXT SESSION:

Dedication

TO WHOM OR WHAT DID YOU DEDICATE THIS CLASS?
(TURN TO PAGE 18 AND ADD YOUR ANSWER TO YOUR DEDICATION LOG.)

Notes and Takeaways

Self-Review

One a scale of 1 to 5 (low to high), rate the following areas of your performance during this session:

FOCUS: 1 2 3 4 5

EVENNESS
OF BREATH: 1 2 3 4 5

BALANCE: 1 2 3 4 5

STRENGTH: 1 2 3 4 5

ENERGY
LEVEL: 1 2 3 4 5

ATTITUDE: 1 2 3 4 5

DATE   /   /   TIME   -

☐ **Group Class Practice**

☐ **Home Practice and/or Private Instruction**

NAME OF STUDIO: ⓞⓡ   IN WHAT ROOM/SPACE DID YOU PRACTICE?

NAME OF TEACHER:

TEACHER RATING (CIRCLE ONE): A+ A A- B C D F

CLASS LEVEL:

☐ BEGINNER ☐ INTERMEDIATE ☐ ADVANCED

CROWD LEVEL: ① ② ③ ④ ⑤
            NOT CROWDED ▸ CROWDED

TEMPERATURE: ☐ HEATED ☐ UNHEATED

ON WHAT PART OF THE BODY DID YOU FOCUS DURING THIS SESSION?

☐ ABDOMINALS   ☐ HIPS
☐ BACK   ☐ BUTTOCKS
☐ SHOULDERS   ☐ LEGS
☐ ARMS   ☐ ANKLES/FEET
☐ WRISTS/HANDS   ☐ OTHER:

Session Details

WHAT STYLE DID YOU PRACTICE DURING THIS SESSION?

☐ ANUSARA   ☐ KRIPALU
☐ ASHTANGA   ☐ KUNDALINI
☐ BIKRAM   ☐ POWER
☐ IYENGAR   ☐ RESTORATIVE
☐ JIVAMUKTI   ☐ VINIYOGA
                 ☐ OTHER:

WHAT TOOLS DID YOU HAVE ON HAND?

☐ MAT   ☐ STRAP
☐ WATER BOTTLE   ☐ BLANKET
☐ TOWEL   ☐ BOLSTER PILLOW
☐ BLOCK   ☐ OTHER:

SOUND ACCOMPANIMENT: ☐ NO MUSIC ☐ MUSIC

FAVORITE TRACK FROM TODAY'S SESSION
(TURN TO PAGE 20 AND ADD THE SONG TO YOUR YOGA SOUNDTRACK.)

Overall Session Rating

PACE OF FLOW: ① ② ③ ④ ⑤

DYNAMISM OF SEQUENCING: ① ② ③ ④ ⑤

DIFFICULTY: ① ② ③ ④ ⑤

POSES INCLUDED IN TODAY'S SEQUENCING:

☐ STANDING POSES   ☐ FORWARD BENDS
☐ BALANCING POSES   ☐ BACKBENDS
☐ SEATED POSES   ☐ INVERSIONS
☐ ABDOMINAL STRENGTHENERS ☐ RESTING POSES
☐ TWISTS

FAVORITE POSE OF TODAY'S SESSION:

MOST CHALLENGING POSE:

POSE YOU HADN'T TRIED BEFORE TODAY:

POSE IN WHICH YOU SHOWED THE MOST IMPROVEMENT:

POSE YOU'D LIKE TO WORK ON IN THE NEXT SESSION:

Dedication

TO WHOM OR WHAT DID YOU DEDICATE THIS CLASS?
(TURN TO PAGE 18 AND ADD YOUR ANSWER TO YOUR DEDICATION LOG.)

Notes and Takeaways

Self-Review

One a scale of 1 to 5 (low to high), rate the following areas of your performance during this session:

FOCUS: 1 2 3 4 5

EVENNESS
OF BREATH: 1 2 3 4 5

BALANCE: 1 2 3 4 5

STRENGTH: 1 2 3 4 5

ENERGY
LEVEL: 1 2 3 4 5

ATTITUDE: 1 2 3 4 5

DATE / / **TIME** -

☐ **Group Class Practice**

☐ **Home Practice and/or Private Instruction**

(OR)

NAME OF STUDIO:

IN WHAT ROOM/SPACE DID YOU PRACTICE?

NAME OF TEACHER:

TEACHER RATING (CIRCLE ONE): A+ A A- B C D F

CLASS LEVEL:
☐ BEGINNER ☐ INTERMEDIATE ☐ ADVANCED

CROWD LEVEL: 1 2 3 4 5
NOT CROWDED ▸ CROWDED

TEMPERATURE: ☐ HEATED ☐ UNHEATED

ON WHAT PART OF THE BODY DID YOU FOCUS DURING THIS SESSION?
☐ ABDOMINALS ☐ HIPS
☐ BACK ☐ BUTTOCKS
☐ SHOULDERS ☐ LEGS
☐ ARMS ☐ ANKLES/FEET
☐ WRISTS/HANDS ☐ OTHER:

Session Details

WHAT STYLE DID YOU PRACTICE DURING THIS SESSION?
☐ ANUSARA ☐ KRIPALU
☐ ASHTANGA ☐ KUNDALINI
☐ BIKRAM ☐ POWER
☐ IYENGAR ☐ RESTORATIVE
☐ JIVAMUKTI ☐ VINIYOGA
☐ OTHER:

WHAT TOOLS DID YOU HAVE ON HAND?
☐ MAT ☐ STRAP
☐ WATER BOTTLE ☐ BLANKET
☐ TOWEL ☐ BOLSTER PILLOW
☐ BLOCK ☐ OTHER:

SOUND ACCOMPANIMENT: ☐ NO MUSIC ☐ MUSIC

FAVORITE TRACK FROM TODAY'S SESSION
(TURN TO PAGE 20 AND ADD THE SONG TO YOUR YOGA SOUNDTRACK.)

Overall Session Rating

PACE OF FLOW: 1 2 3 4 5

DYNAMISM OF SEQUENCING: 1 2 3 4 5

DIFFICULTY: 1 2 3 4 5

POSES INCLUDED IN TODAY'S SEQUENCING:
☐ STANDING POSES ☐ FORWARD BENDS
☐ BALANCING POSES ☐ BACKBENDS
☐ SEATED POSES ☐ INVERSIONS
☐ ABDOMINAL STRENGTHENERS ☐ RESTING POSES
☐ TWISTS

FAVORITE POSE OF TODAY'S SESSION:

MOST CHALLENGING POSE:

POSE YOU HADN'T TRIED BEFORE TODAY:

POSE IN WHICH YOU SHOWED THE MOST IMPROVEMENT:

POSE YOU'D LIKE TO WORK ON IN THE NEXT SESSION:

Dedication

TO WHOM OR WHAT DID YOU DEDICATE THIS CLASS?
(TURN TO PAGE 18 AND ADD YOUR ANSWER TO YOUR DEDICATION LOG.)

Notes and Takeaways

Self-Review

One a scale of 1 to 5 (low to high), rate the following areas of your performance during this session:

FOCUS: 1 2 3 4 5

EVENNESS
OF BREATH: 1 2 3 4 5

BALANCE: 1 2 3 4 5

STRENGTH: 1 2 3 4 5

ENERGY
LEVEL: 1 2 3 4 5

ATTITUDE: 1 2 3 4 5

DATE / / **TIME** -

☐ **Group Class Practice**

☐ **Home Practice and/or Private Instruction**

NAME OF STUDIO:

(OR)

IN WHAT ROOM/SPACE DID YOU PRACTICE?

NAME OF TEACHER:

TEACHER RATING (CIRCLE ONE): A+ A A- B C D F

CLASS LEVEL:
☐ BEGINNER ☐ INTERMEDIATE ☐ ADVANCED

CROWD LEVEL: ①·②·③·④·⑤
NOT CROWDED ▶ CROWDED

TEMPERATURE: ☐ HEATED ☐ UNHEATED

ON WHAT PART OF THE BODY DID YOU FOCUS DURING THIS SESSION?

☐ ABDOMINALS   ☐ HIPS
☐ BACK   ☐ BUTTOCKS
☐ SHOULDERS   ☐ LEGS
☐ ARMS   ☐ ANKLES/FEET
☐ WRISTS/HANDS ☐ OTHER:

Session Details

WHAT STYLE DID YOU PRACTICE DURING THIS SESSION?

☐ ANUSARA   ☐ KRIPALU
☐ ASHTANGA   ☐ KUNDALINI
☐ BIKRAM   ☐ POWER
☐ IYENGAR   ☐ RESTORATIVE
☐ JIVAMUKTI   ☐ VINIYOGA
               ☐ OTHER:

WHAT TOOLS DID YOU HAVE ON HAND?

☐ MAT   ☐ STRAP
☐ WATER BOTTLE   ☐ BLANKET
☐ TOWEL   ☐ BOLSTER PILLOW
☐ BLOCK   ☐ OTHER:

SOUND ACCOMPANIMENT: ☐ NO MUSIC ☐ MUSIC

FAVORITE TRACK FROM TODAY'S SESSION

(TURN TO PAGE 20 AND ADD THE SONG TO YOUR YOGA SOUNDTRACK.)

Overall Session Rating

PACE OF FLOW: ①·②·③·④·⑤

DYNAMISM OF SEQUENCING: ①·②·③·④·⑤

DIFFICULTY: ①·②·③·④·⑤

POSES INCLUDED IN TODAY'S SEQUENCING:

☐ STANDING POSES   ☐ FORWARD BENDS
☐ BALANCING POSES   ☐ BACKBENDS
☐ SEATED POSES   ☐ INVERSIONS
☐ ABDOMINAL STRENGTHENERS   ☐ RESTING POSES
☐ TWISTS

FAVORITE POSE OF TODAY'S SESSION:

MOST CHALLENGING POSE:

POSE YOU HADN'T TRIED BEFORE TODAY:

POSE IN WHICH YOU SHOWED THE MOST IMPROVEMENT:

POSE YOU'D LIKE TO WORK ON IN THE NEXT SESSION:

Dedication

TO WHOM OR WHAT DID YOU DEDICATE THIS CLASS?
(TURN TO PAGE 18 AND ADD YOUR ANSWER TO YOUR DEDICATION LOG.)

Notes and Takeaways

Self-Review

One a scale of 1 to 5 (low to high), rate the following areas of your performance during this session:

FOCUS:	1	2	3	4	5
EVENNESS OF BREATH:	1	2	3	4	5
BALANCE:	1	2	3	4	5
STRENGTH:	1	2	3	4	5
ENERGY LEVEL:	1	2	3	4	5
ATTITUDE:	1	2	3	4	5

DATE   /   /   **TIME**   -

☐ Group Class Practice

☐ Home Practice and/or Private Instruction

(OR)

NAME OF STUDIO:

IN WHAT ROOM/SPACE DID YOU PRACTICE?

NAME OF TEACHER:

TEACHER RATING (CIRCLE ONE): A+ A A- B C D F

ON WHAT PART OF THE BODY DID YOU FOCUS DURING THIS SESSION?

CLASS LEVEL:

☐ BEGINNER   ☐ INTERMEDIATE   ☐ ADVANCED

CROWD LEVEL: 1 2 3 4 5

NOT CROWDED ▸ CROWDED

TEMPERATURE: ☐ HEATED   ☐ UNHEATED

☐ ABDOMINALS   ☐ HIPS
☐ BACK   ☐ BUTTOCKS
☐ SHOULDERS   ☐ LEGS
☐ ARMS   ☐ ANKLES/FEET
☐ WRISTS/HANDS   ☐ OTHER:

Session Details

WHAT STYLE DID YOU PRACTICE DURING THIS SESSION?

☐ ANUSARA   ☐ KRIPALU
☐ ASHTANGA   ☐ KUNDALINI
☐ BIKRAM   ☐ POWER
☐ IYENGAR   ☐ RESTORATIVE
☐ JIVAMUKTI   ☐ VINIYOGA
                ☐ OTHER:

WHAT TOOLS DID YOU HAVE ON HAND?

☐ MAT   ☐ STRAP
☐ WATER BOTTLE   ☐ BLANKET
☐ TOWEL   ☐ BOLSTER PILLOW
☐ BLOCK   ☐ OTHER:

SOUND ACCOMPANIMENT: ☐ NO MUSIC   ☐ MUSIC

FAVORITE TRACK FROM TODAY'S SESSION

(TURN TO PAGE 20 AND ADD THE SONG TO YOUR YOGA SOUNDTRACK.)

Overall Session Rating

PACE OF FLOW: 1 2 3 4 5

DYNAMISM OF SEQUENCING: 1 2 3 4 5

DIFFICULTY: 1 2 3 4 5

POSES INCLUDED IN TODAY'S SEQUENCING:

☐ STANDING POSES   ☐ FORWARD BENDS
☐ BALANCING POSES   ☐ BACKBENDS
☐ SEATED POSES   ☐ INVERSIONS
☐ ABDOMINAL STRENGTHENERS   ☐ RESTING POSES
☐ TWISTS

FAVORITE POSE OF TODAY'S SESSION:

MOST CHALLENGING POSE:

POSE YOU HADN'T TRIED BEFORE TODAY:

POSE IN WHICH YOU SHOWED THE MOST IMPROVEMENT:

POSE YOU'D LIKE TO WORK ON IN THE NEXT SESSION:

Dedication

TO WHOM OR WHAT DID YOU DEDICATE THIS CLASS?
(TURN TO PAGE 18 AND ADD YOUR ANSWER TO YOUR DEDICATION LOG.)

Notes and Takeaways

Self-Review

One a scale of 1 to 5 (low to high), rate the following areas of your performance during this session:

FOCUS:	1 2 3 4 5
EVENNESS OF BREATH:	1 2 3 4 5
BALANCE:	1 2 3 4 5
STRENGTH:	1 2 3 4 5
ENERGY LEVEL:	1 2 3 4 5
ATTITUDE:	1 2 3 4 5

DATE   /   /   TIME   -

☐ **Group Class Practice**

NAME OF STUDIO:

NAME OF TEACHER:

TEACHER RATING (CIRCLE ONE): A+ A A- B C D F

CLASS LEVEL:
☐ BEGINNER   ☐ INTERMEDIATE   ☐ ADVANCED

CROWD LEVEL: 1 2 3 4 5
             NOT CROWDED ▸ CROWDED

TEMPERATURE: ☐ HEATED   ☐ UNHEATED

(OR)

☐ **Home Practice and/or Private Instruction**

IN WHAT ROOM/SPACE DID YOU PRACTICE?

ON WHAT PART OF THE BODY DID YOU FOCUS DURING THIS SESSION?

☐ ABDOMINALS   ☐ HIPS
☐ BACK   ☐ BUTTOCKS
☐ SHOULDERS   ☐ LEGS
☐ ARMS   ☐ ANKLES/FEET
☐ WRISTS/HANDS   ☐ OTHER:

Session Details

WHAT STYLE DID YOU PRACTICE DURING THIS SESSION?

☐ ANUSARA   ☐ KRIPALU
☐ ASHTANGA   ☐ KUNDALINI
☐ BIKRAM   ☐ POWER
☐ IYENGAR   ☐ RESTORATIVE
☐ JIVAMUKTI   ☐ VINIYOGA
               ☐ OTHER:

WHAT TOOLS DID YOU HAVE ON HAND?

☐ MAT   ☐ STRAP
☐ WATER BOTTLE   ☐ BLANKET
☐ TOWEL   ☐ BOLSTER PILLOW
☐ BLOCK   ☐ OTHER:

SOUND ACCOMPANIMENT: ☐ NO MUSIC   ☐ MUSIC

FAVORITE TRACK FROM TODAY'S SESSION
(TURN TO PAGE 20 AND ADD THE SONG TO YOUR YOGA SOUNDTRACK.)

Overall Session Rating

PACE OF FLOW: 1 2 3 4 5

DYNAMISM OF SEQUENCING: 1 2 3 4 5

DIFFICULTY: 1 2 3 4 5

POSES INCLUDED IN TODAY'S SEQUENCING:

☐ STANDING POSES   ☐ FORWARD BENDS
☐ BALANCING POSES   ☐ BACKBENDS
☐ SEATED POSES   ☐ INVERSIONS
☐ ABDOMINAL STRENGTHENERS   ☐ RESTING POSES
☐ TWISTS

FAVORITE POSE OF TODAY'S SESSION:

MOST CHALLENGING POSE: .

POSE YOU HADN'T TRIED BEFORE TODAY:

POSE IN WHICH YOU SHOWED THE MOST IMPROVEMENT:

POSE YOU'D LIKE TO WORK ON IN THE NEXT SESSION:

Dedication

TO WHOM OR WHAT DID YOU DEDICATE THIS CLASS?
(TURN TO PAGE 18 AND ADD YOUR ANSWER TO YOUR DEDICATION LOG.)

Notes and Takeaways

Self-Review

One a scale of 1 to 5 (low to high), rate the following areas of your performance during this session:

FOCUS: 1 2 3 4 5

EVENNESS
OF BREATH: 1 2 3 4 5

BALANCE: 1 2 3 4 5

STRENGTH: 1 2 3 4 5

ENERGY
LEVEL: 1 2 3 4 5

ATTITUDE: 1 2 3 4 5

Yoga Session (43)

DATE / / **TIME** -

☐ **Group Class Practice**　　　☐ **Home Practice and/or Private Instruction**

NAME OF STUDIO:

NAME OF TEACHER:

TEACHER RATING (CIRCLE ONE): A+ A A- B C D F

CLASS LEVEL:
☐ BEGINNER ☐ INTERMEDIATE ☐ ADVANCED

CROWD LEVEL: 1 2 3 4 5
　　　　　NOT CROWDED ▶ CROWDED

TEMPERATURE: ☐ HEATED ☐ UNHEATED

(OR) IN WHAT ROOM/SPACE DID YOU PRACTICE?

ON WHAT PART OF THE BODY DID YOU FOCUS DURING THIS SESSION?
☐ ABDOMINALS ☐ HIPS
☐ BACK ☐ BUTTOCKS
☐ SHOULDERS ☐ LEGS
☐ ARMS ☐ ANKLES/FEET
☐ WRISTS/HANDS ☐ OTHER:

Session Details

WHAT STYLE DID YOU PRACTICE DURING THIS SESSION?
☐ ANUSARA ☐ KRIPALU
☐ ASHTANGA ☐ KUNDALINI
☐ BIKRAM ☐ POWER
☐ IYENGAR ☐ RESTORATIVE
☐ JIVAMUKTI ☐ VINIYOGA
　　　　 ☐ OTHER:

WHAT TOOLS DID YOU HAVE ON HAND?
☐ MAT ☐ STRAP
☐ WATER BOTTLE ☐ BLANKET
☐ TOWEL ☐ BOLSTER PILLOW
☐ BLOCK ☐ OTHER:

SOUND ACCOMPANIMENT: ☐ NO MUSIC ☐ MUSIC

FAVORITE TRACK FROM TODAY'S SESSION
(TURN TO PAGE 29 AND ADD THE SONG TO YOUR YOGA SOUNDTRACK.)

Overall Session Rating

PACE OF FLOW: 1 2 3 4 5

DYNAMISM OF SEQUENCING: 1 2 3 4 5

DIFFICULTY: 1 2 3 4 5

POSES INCLUDED IN TODAY'S SEQUENCING:
☐ STANDING POSES ☐ FORWARD BENDS
☐ BALANCING POSES ☐ BACKBENDS
☐ SEATED POSES ☐ INVERSIONS
☐ ABDOMINAL STRENGTHENERS ☐ RESTING POSES
☐ TWISTS

FAVORITE POSE OF TODAY'S SESSION:

MOST CHALLENGING POSE:

POSE YOU HADN'T TRIED BEFORE TODAY:

POSE IN WHICH YOU SHOWED THE MOST IMPROVEMENT:

POSE YOU'D LIKE TO WORK ON IN THE NEXT SESSION:

Dedication

TO WHOM OR WHAT DID YOU DEDICATE THIS CLASS?
(TURN TO PAGE 18 AND ADD YOUR ANSWER TO YOUR DEDICATION LOG.)

Notes and Takeaways

Self-Review

One a scale of 1 to 5 (low to high), rate the following areas of your performance during this session:

FOCUS: 1 2 3 4 5

EVENNESS
OF BREATH: 1 2 3 4 5

BALANCE: 1 2 3 4 5

STRENGTH: 1 2 3 4 5

ENERGY
LEVEL: 1 2 3 4 5

ATTITUDE: 1 2 3 4 5

DATE   /   /   TIME   -

☐ **Group Class Practice**

☐ **Home Practice and/or Private Instruction**

NAME OF STUDIO:

(OR)   IN WHAT ROOM/SPACE DID YOU PRACTICE?

NAME OF TEACHER:

TEACHER RATING (CIRCLE ONE): A+ A A- B C D F

CLASS LEVEL:

☐ BEGINNER   ☐ INTERMEDIATE   ☐ ADVANCED

CROWD LEVEL: 1 2 3 4 5
              NOT CROWDED → CROWDED

TEMPERATURE: ☐ HEATED   ☐ UNHEATED

ON WHAT PART OF THE BODY DID YOU FOCUS DURING THIS SESSION?

☐ ABDOMINALS   ☐ HIPS
☐ BACK   ☐ BUTTOCKS
☐ SHOULDERS   ☐ LEGS
☐ ARMS   ☐ ANKLES/FEET
☐ WRISTS/HANDS ☐ OTHER:

Session Details

WHAT STYLE DID YOU PRACTICE DURING THIS SESSION?

☐ ANUSARA   ☐ KRIPALU
☐ ASHTANGA   ☐ KUNDALINI
☐ BIKRAM   ☐ POWER
☐ IYENGAR   ☐ RESTORATIVE
☐ JIVAMUKTI   ☐ VINIYOGA
                 ☐ OTHER:

WHAT TOOLS DID YOU HAVE ON HAND?

☐ MAT   ☐ STRAP
☐ WATER BOTTLE   ☐ BLANKET
☐ TOWEL   ☐ BOLSTER PILLOW
☐ BLOCK   ☐ OTHER:

SOUND ACCOMPANIMENT: ☐ NO MUSIC   ☐ MUSIC

FAVORITE TRACK FROM TODAY'S SESSION
(TURN TO PAGE 20 AND ADD THE SONG TO YOUR YOGA SOUNDTRACK.)

Overall Session Rating

PACE OF FLOW: 1 2 3 4 5

DYNAMISM OF SEQUENCING: 1 2 3 4 5

DIFFICULTY: 1 2 3 4 5

POSES INCLUDED IN TODAY'S SEQUENCING:

☐ STANDING POSES   ☐ FORWARD BENDS
☐ BALANCING POSES   ☐ BACKBENDS
☐ SEATED POSES   ☐ INVERSIONS
☐ ABDOMINAL   ☐ RESTING POSES
  STRENGTHENERS
☐ TWISTS

FAVORITE POSE OF TODAY'S SESSION:

MOST CHALLENGING POSE:

POSE YOU HADN'T TRIED BEFORE TODAY:

POSE IN WHICH YOU SHOWED THE MOST IMPROVEMENT:

POSE YOU'D LIKE TO WORK ON IN THE NEXT SESSION:

Dedication

TO WHOM OR WHAT DID YOU DEDICATE THIS CLASS?
(TURN TO PAGE 18 AND ADD YOUR ANSWER TO YOUR DEDICATION LOG.)

Notes and Takeaways

Self-Review

One a scale of 1 to 5 (low to high), rate the following areas of your performance during this session:

FOCUS:	1	2	3	4	5
EVENNESS OF BREATH:	1	2	3	4	5
BALANCE:	1	2	3	4	5
STRENGTH:	1	2	3	4	5
ENERGY LEVEL:	1	2	3	4	5
ATTITUDE:	1	2	3	4	5

Yoga Session (45)

DATE   /   /   TIME   -

☐ **Group Class Practice**

☐ **Home Practice and/or Private Instruction**

NAME OF STUDIO:

(OR)   IN WHAT ROOM/SPACE DID YOU PRACTICE?

NAME OF TEACHER:

TEACHER RATING (CIRCLE ONE): A+ A A- B C D F

CLASS LEVEL:

☐ BEGINNER   ☐ INTERMEDIATE   ☐ ADVANCED

CROWD LEVEL: 1 2 3 4 5

TEMPERATURE: ☐ HEATED   ☐ UNHEATED

ON WHAT PART OF THE BODY DID YOU FOCUS DURING THIS SESSION?

☐ ABDOMINALS   ☐ HIPS
☐ BACK   ☐ BUTTOCKS
☐ SHOULDERS   ☐ LEGS
☐ ARMS   ☐ ANKLES/FEET
☐ WRISTS/HANDS   ☐ OTHER:

Session Details

WHAT STYLE DID YOU PRACTICE DURING THIS SESSION?

☐ ANUSARA   ☐ KRIPALU
☐ ASHTANGA   ☐ KUNDALINI
☐ BIKRAM   ☐ POWER
☐ IYENGAR   ☐ RESTORATIVE
☐ JIVAMUKTI   ☐ VINIYOGA
                 ☐ OTHER:

WHAT TOOLS DID YOU HAVE ON HAND?

☐ MAT   ☐ STRAP
☐ WATER BOTTLE   ☐ BLANKET
☐ TOWEL   ☐ BOLSTER PILLOW
☐ BLOCK   ☐ OTHER:

SOUND ACCOMPANIMENT: ☐ NO MUSIC   ☐ MUSIC

FAVORITE TRACK FROM TODAY'S SESSION

Overall Session Rating

PACE OF FLOW: 1 2 3 4 5

DYNAMISM OF SEQUENCING: 1 2 3 4 5

DIFFICULTY: 1 2 3 4 5

POSES INCLUDED IN TODAY'S SEQUENCING:

☐ STANDING POSES   ☐ FORWARD BENDS
☐ BALANCING POSES   ☐ BACKBENDS
☐ SEATED POSES   ☐ INVERSIONS
☐ ABDOMINAL
  STRENGTHENERS   ☐ RESTING POSES
☐ TWISTS

FAVORITE POSE OF TODAY'S SESSION:

MOST CHALLENGING POSE:

POSE YOU HADN'T TRIED BEFORE TODAY:

POSE IN WHICH YOU SHOWED THE MOST IMPROVEMENT:

POSE YOU'D LIKE TO WORK ON IN THE NEXT SESSION:

Dedication

TO WHOM OR WHAT DID YOU DEDICATE THIS CLASS?
(TURN TO PAGE 18 AND ADD YOUR ANSWER TO YOUR DEDICATION LOG.)

Notes and Takeaways

Self-Review

One a scale of 1 to 5 (low to high), rate the following areas of your performance during this session:

FOCUS: 1 2 3 4 5

EVENNESS
OF BREATH: 1 2 3 4 5

BALANCE: 1 2 3 4 5

STRENGTH: 1 2 3 4 5

ENERGY
LEVEL: 1 2 3 4 5

ATTITUDE: 1 2 3 4 5

Yoga
Reference
Guide

A Brief History of Yoga

The history of yoga is a complex web of branches and schools that twist and turn, leading to what is considered today's modern yoga. No one can pinpoint precisely when yoga was invented, but here's what we do know: Yoga hails from India. The language of yoga is called Sanskrit, an ancient priestly tongue. A pose is called an *asana*, based on the Sanskrit word for "seat." The yoga lifestyle has changed quite a bit since ancient times, when yogis lived in secluded caves or forests and practiced ways to master their bodies, such as stopping their heartbeat. But the essence of yoga remains the same, as does the ultimate goal: to find harmony with yourself and the world.

The Ancient Age
(3000 BCE–300 BCE)

Some scholars believe the yoga tradition began as early as 5,000 years ago, linking its origins to a soapstone seal, which was excavated in the early 1900s, that had humanlike figures carved in shapes that looked like yoga poses. Others believe yoga is 2,500 years old, which is when it was first mentioned in an ancient text. Still others believe that yoga originated during the Vedic Age in India, when people focused on ritual, poetry, and transcending the mind through intense focus. During this time, holy men and women were said to have magical powers and practiced strenuous physical feats to overcome the body, which they considered an obstacle to enlightenment. These early yogis were committed to understanding their relationship with the divine, a core idea that is found in many schools of yoga today, thousands of years later. Over time, the focus shifted from study and rituals toward self-understanding through direct experience. The body was no longer considered an obstacle; rather, it was seen as a means to finding freedom.

The Classical Age
(300 BCE–500 CE)

In yoga's Classical Age, which also took place in India, yoga came to be seen as a spiritual philosophy that could help people reach their full human potential. Finding freedom wasn't so much about uniting with some great spirit in the sky, but about awakening to their own authentic self. It's known as the Classical Age because during this time, six classical philosophies were established, one of which is Patanjali's yoga. Patanjali was a sage who lived at the dawn on the first millennium. He wrote *The Yoga Sutra*, an authoritative text of the Classical Age containing a set of guidelines called the Eight-Limbed Path (see page 144) that serves as a template for some modern-day yoga schools. During this era, the emphasis of the practice was on meditation rather than on yoga's physical poses.

The Modern Age
(1893–present)

Modern yoga as we know it gained traction in the late 1800s after a few individual Indian yogis shared teachings of Eastern philosophy with Western audiences. Among those was Swami Vivekananda, a Hindu monk who gave an influential speech at the World's Parliament of Religions in Chicago in 1893. Over the next century, more Indian teachers came to America, including B.K.S. Iyengar, Pattabhi Jois, Indra Devi, and T.K.V. Desikachar. These teachers, all students of a great Indian master called Krishnamacharya, went on to create the major styles practiced by today's yogis. Another Indian teacher, Paramahansa Yogananda, came to Boston in 1920 and founded the Self-Realization Fellowship. His book, *Autobiography of a Yogi*, is a wildly popular spiritual classic.

By the 1960s, yoga had taken hold in Western counterculture. An Indian guru named Swami Satchidananda gave the opening speech at Woodstock in 1969, while the Beatles started traveling to India to study with a guru named Maharishi Mahesh Yogi. Ram Dass wrote a famous book called *Be Here Now* that heralded in the age of spiritual seekers. B.K.S. Iyengar wrote *Light on Yoga* which is considered to be the definitive manual on modern yoga. By the 1990s, yoga's popularity had fully transitioned from counterculture to the mainstream, where it thrives today.

The Branches of Yoga

Whether it's rigorous exercise that opens one's heart, or music, or service to others, there's a branch of yoga for everyone.

Here are the modern forms of today's most relevant branches:

Bhakti Yoga: The Yoga of Devotion

Purpose: To develop a personal relationship with the divine, however one chooses to define it

Hatha Yoga: The Yoga of Physical Exercise

Purpose: To purify the body and mind through yoga poses

Jnana Yoga: The Yoga of Wisdom

Purpose: To seek and understand the truth

Karma Yoga: The Yoga of Service

Purpose: To selflessly help others

Mantra Yoga: The Yoga of Sound

Purpose: To focus the mind by repeating a chosen mantra or sound

Raja Yoga: The Yoga of Meditation

Purpose: To experience moments of peace and clarity through quiet contemplation

Yoga Styles

When yoga hit the West in the late nineteenth century, a natural evolution occurred. Teachers trained by Indian masters began taking what they had learned and making it their own. Some instructors opened schools that followed closely in their particular lineage, while others used their knowledge as a starting point to develop their own creative styles. These days, there's a wide range of yoga styles suited to all personalities and skill levels, with variations in speed, levels of exertion, purposes, benefits, and environment (such as temperature of the room and noise level, for example).

Today's most popular styles include:

· Anusara Yoga

· Ashtanga Yoga

· Bikram Yoga

· Iyengar Yoga

· Jivamukti Yoga

· Kripalu Yoga

· Kundalini Yoga

· Power Yoga

· Restorative Yoga

· Viniyoga

Anusara Yoga

Anusara yoga presents the idea that, when practiced with proper alignment and intention, the poses can help one connect with inner joy, creativity, playfulness, and one's full potential. Rather than focusing on what needs to be fixed or corrected, Anusara teachers focus on the thriving goodness within and around us and seek to help uncover each student's unique, innate beauty. Anusara's Universal Principles of Alignment, which incorporate yoga philosophy and physical alignment techniques, are applied to the teaching of each pose. Classes include an opening invocation, a heart-opening theme, a flowing sequence chosen from a selection of more than 250 poses, and a final relaxation period.

Ashtanga Yoga

Ashtanga yoga, founded by K. Pattabhi Jois (1915–2009), features flowing movements called *vinyasas* that connect breath with movement. When done correctly, the blood circulates freely, creating internal heat and sweating, which is believed to purify the body and calm the mind. Sometimes referred to as Ashtanga Vinyasa Yoga, this style follows a universal sequence that students gradually learn from their teacher as they progress in skill and ability. Classes open with Sun Salutations (see page 148), followed by standing poses, seated poses, backbends, inversions, and finally a relaxation pose. Flow yoga and vinyasa yoga are variations of Ashtanga yoga.

Bikram Yoga

Bikram yoga, founded by Bikram Choudhury (b. 1946), is a standardized series of twenty-six poses practiced in a room heated to 105°F/40°C. The heat is believed to release toxins, improve circulation, and loosen up muscles. Because of the heat, it's recommended that you dress lightly and bring a towel and a bottle of water. The practice starts and ends with breathing exercises and includes standing poses, backbends, seated poses, and twists. Each pose is done twice, and proceeds in a fixed order. It's often called Hot Yoga when there is some deviation from Bikram's prescribed sequence.

Iyengar Yoga

Iyengar yoga was founded by B.K.S. Iyengar (b. 1918), who considered the body to be a vehicle toward a spiritual path. This style emphasizes precise alignment, anatomy, and sequencing of the poses in a very specific order. Classes are conducted like an in-depth workshop, focusing on only a few poses, hands-on adjustments, and holding demonstrations in the center of the room. Iyengar yoga encourages the use of props like blocks, chairs, blankets, and bolsters to promote relaxation, proper alignment, and opening the body in a safe way. Those who are sensitive to injury, or are healing from a specific injury, find Iyengar useful because of the careful instructions, attention to body mechanics, and thoughtful modifications of the poses to suit individual needs and comfort preferences.

Jivamukti Yoga

Jivamukti yoga, founded in New York City by Sharon Gannon and David Life in 1986, is a rigorous form of flowing yoga. Energetic Jivamukti classes include Sun Salutations, poses, chanting, music, relaxation, and meditation. Some classes open with a theme that is woven throughout the class, and there is an emphasis on alignment and hands-on adjustment. Loosely translated from Sanskrit, *jivan mukti* means "liberation while living." The founders' philosophy centers around five tenets: kindness, devotion, meditation, music, and studying yoga scripture. They encourage practitioners to bring yoga philosophy off the mat and into their daily lives and to live in a kind and compassionate way.

Kripalu Yoga

Kripalu yoga was founded by Amrit Desai (b. 1932), a native of India who was inspired by Swami Kripalvananda (1913–1981), after whom the practice is named. With a focus on bringing awareness to poses, breathwork, and meditation, Kripalu yoga encourages healing, psychological growth, spirituality, and creativity. By focusing on staying in the present moment while on the mat, this style encourages deepening your spiritual attunement, self-awareness, and empathy. It combines a slow-moving yet challenging class with a meditative awareness. Kripalu employs an approach referred to as BRFWA: breathe, relax, feel, watch, and allow.

Kundalini Yoga

Kundalini yoga practices—including breathing, poses, hand positions, chanting, and meditation—are designed to awaken the latent energy that sits at the base of the spine so that one can experience a higher consciousness. The practices focus on balancing the glandular and nervous systems for physical, mental, and spiritual health. A chant often heard in a Kundalini yoga class is *Sat Nam*, which means "truth is my identity." Kundalini yoga, as inspired by Yogi Bhajan (1929-2004), encourages teachers and practitioners to wear white clothing to nourish light and divinity.

Power Yoga

Power yoga is an overarching term for an athletic style of yoga that is popular in a gym setting as well as in studios. Its roots are in Ashtanga yoga. Poses are linked together by a *chaturanga* (four-limbed staff) pose (see page 149), and movements flow swiftly for an often sweaty cardio workout, likely accompanied by upbeat music. Variations of Power yoga are Power Vinyasa, Power Vinyasa Flow, and Dynamic Yoga.

Restorative Yoga

Restorative yoga is designed to counter stress by triggering the para-sympathetic nervous system, which calms the body and lowers heart rate and blood pressure. Restorative yoga poses often incorporate props such as bolsters, blocks, and blankets that completely support the body, allowing it to relax and drop deeply into a stress-free state. Each pose requires time for the practitioner to arrange the body and adjust props until they arrive in a position of complete comfort. Once there, they lie still for up to twenty minutes. Restorative yoga was popularized by Judith Hanson Lasater—a physical therapist, yoga teacher, and scholar—in the 1990s.

Viniyoga

Viniyoga is useful for all kinds of yogis and is often recommended for people with injuries or illness because it's highly adaptable to one's needs. The practice includes poses, breathwork, meditation, chanting, and other methods designed to transform the body and mind. In a Viniyoga class, one might move in and out of the same pose repeatedly, making slight modifications while also focusing on the breath. Viniyoga was shaped by Gary Kraftsow (b. 1955), who based the practice on the teachings of Krishnamacharya (1888–1989) and T.K.V. Desikachar (b. 1938).

What Is Hatha Yoga?

Hatha yoga refers specifically to the physical aspect of yoga. The word *hatha* in Sanskrit means "force," which can describe the strengthening movements of the body during a yoga class. Historically, physical movement was just one small part of the larger yoga tradition, but today the physical exercises known as Hatha yoga are what many recognize as modern yoga. Classes described as "hatha" often blend a few different styles rather than emphasizing just one.

What Is Vinyasa Yoga?

Some modern yoga classes are referred to as "Vinyasa yoga," which means that poses are linked together with flowing movements and often linked to the breath. Vinyasa also refers to carefully thought-out sequencing, with one pose preparing the body for the next. Think of Vinyasa as a graceful dance, with the same moves being repeated continuously.

Yoga Philosophy

The Eight-Limbed Path

Modern-day yoga is known for its physical poses, but the poses are just one step on what the ancient yogis believed was a path to enlightenment. The Eight-Limbed Path—outlined by prolific sage Patanjali (born between 300 BCE and AD 200) in his collection of writings called *The Yoga Sutra*—is a system of moral and ethical guidelines and practices including yoga poses that lead the yogi to a peaceful life. Thousands of years after the Eight Limbs were first recorded, many yoga schools still use them as the foundation of their practice, while individual yogis find that they apply seamlessly to everyday living, off the mat.

The eight limbs of the Eight-Limbed Path—like the limbs of a tree—are integrally linked to each other, proceeding in a basic order, from external to internal, guiding us toward inner peace. Our journey starts with the first limb, or *yama*, which consists of five principles that help make us aware of how we see and interact with the external world. Next, we arrive at *niyama*, the second limb, which also consists of five principles. The *niyamas* invite us to look inward and truly get to know ourselves through reflection and self-study. The third and fourth limbs are active, energetic practices. In Patanjali's day, the third limb, or *asana*, meant a comfortable seated position. Today it refers to yoga's physical poses. The fourth limb, *pranayama*, meant a practice of slowing the breath and has since evolved into the various breathing exercises that we know today. Both of these limbs, *asana* and *pranayama*, prepare the body and mind for the three limbs that follow: *pratyahara*, inward focus by withdrawing the five senses; *dharana*, concentration; and *dhyana*, meditation. The eighth and final limb—which is understood to be the ultimate reward—is *samadhi*, described by some as ecstasy and by others more simply as enlightenment, contentment, or inner peace.

Samadhi is a grandiose concept, but Patanjali and the ancient yogis believed it to be achievable by every human being of any means. Indeed, today we might understand *samadhi* to be the natural, blissful reward of being kind to others, nurturing the self, and living in the moment. The following page provides at-a-glance reminders of each limb of the Eight-Limbed Path, followed by closer examinations of the *yamas* and the *niyamas*.

The Eight Limbs

1.
Yama: Universal morality

2.
Niyama: Personal morality

3.
Asana: Physical practices

4.
Pranayama: Breathing practices

5.
Pratyahara: Withdrawal of the senses

6.
Dharana: Concentration

7.
Dhyana: Meditation

8.
Samadhi: Enlightenment

The Five Yamas

Yama is the first limb of yoga's Eight-Limbed Path. Also translated as "restraints," the *yamas* introduce five ethical guidelines that focus on the ways of viewing the external world and interacting with others. The *yamas*, such as telling the truth and not stealing, are considered a foundation of a yoga practice.

1. *Ahimsa*: Nonharming

To practice *ahimsa* means to live a life of nonviolence, avoiding physical, verbal, and emotional abuse of others and one's self. To resist striving for perfection. To release one's self from unrealistic ideals. To adopt a kind, forgiving, and gentle approach to life.

2. *Satya*: Honesty

To practice *satya* means to be straightforward in speech and action. To study one's self closely and identify the roots of dishonest behavior. To correct others' misperceptions of one's character or circumstances. To act in ways that are in harmony with one's inner truth.

3. *Asteya*: Not stealing

To practice *asteya* means to resist the dissatisfaction that can lead to coveting or stealing from another. To be content with one's own belongings and circumstances. To resist comparing one's self to others. To practice gratitude and to cultivate self-acceptance.

4. *Brahmacharya*: Sensual moderation

To practice *brahmacharya* means to practice moderation. To be thoughtful about how one indulges the five senses. To avoid addiction. To reflect on outcomes (good and bad) with the aim of boosting the honesty and integrity of one's actions.

5. *Aparigraha*: Nonpossessiveness

To practice *aparigraha* means to release attachment to material possessions, emotions, and accomplishments. To free one's self from the clinging and worry that accompany attachment. To create room in one's life for fresh possibilities and powerful positive energy. To let go, and in doing so, to welcome in the basic faith that the universe will provide.

The Five Niyamas

Translated as "observances," the *niyamas* are the second limb of Patanjali's Eight-Limbed Path. While the first limb, the *yamas*, addresses the external world and how one relates to others, the *niyamas* deal with the inner world—personal rather than interpersonal guidelines.

1. *Saucha*: Purity

To practice *saucha* means to create and maintain pure energy inside the body and out. To unload possessions and habits that are holding one back. To clear the literal and figurative path to enlightenment.

2. *Santosha*: Contentment

To practice *santosha* means to resist self-doubt. To curb jealousy. To recognize there is not just one way to happiness but a unique path for every human being. To actively accept one's circumstances without fear, judgment, or expectation.

3. *Tapas*: Self-discipline

To practice *tapas* means to persevere. To act with integrity and intention. To cultivate self-reliance and faith that any situation can be endured and any circumstance overcome. To maintain the commitment to self-betterment.

4. *Svadhyaya*: Self-study

To practice *svadhyaya* means to observe patterns in one's thinking and behavior. To tap into the true self. To make decisions that are better aligned with one's individual calling, and in doing so, to live a more authentic life.

5. *Ishvara pranidhana*: Surrender

To practice *ishvara pranidhana* means to release attachments to outcomes. To release one's self from judgments and expectations. To have faith in something outside the self. To liberate the self from the grip of the ego.

Illustrated Yoga Pose Directory

With hundreds of poses to choose from, a yoga practice is infinitely customizable for every skill level, personality, and wellness goal. Yoga poses can be the center of a fitness program or can be an occasional add-on. Individually or grouped together, they can target specific muscles and areas of the body. Strung together into dynamic sequences, they can provide a full-body workout. The following pages present a sampling of some of the most commonly taught yoga poses, ideal for mixing, matching, and modifying to suit anyone's wellness goals.

Sun Salutation

Yoga's classic Sun Salutation (*Surya Namaskar*, in Sanskrit) is a flowing sequence that awakens the body and mind. Do it two times briskly on each side, linking each movement with your breath, for an energizing way to greet the day.

1. Mountain Pose

2. Mountain Pose with Arms Up

3. Standing Forward Bend

4. Lunge (Left Leg Forward)

5. Plank Pose

6. Four-Limbed Staff Pose

7. Upward-Facing Dog

8. Downward-Facing Dog

9. Lunge (Right Leg Forward)

10. Standing Forward Bend

11. Mountain Pose with Arms Up

12. Mountain Pose

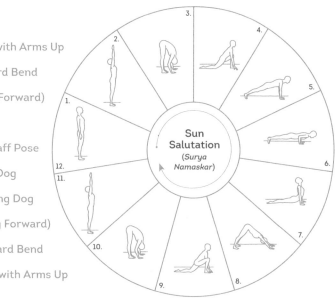

Sun Salutation Poses

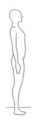

MOUNTAIN POSE
TADASANA
(ta-DA-sah-nah)

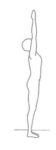

MOUNTAIN POSE WITH ARMS UP

STANDING FORWARD BEND

LUNGE

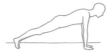

PLANK POSE

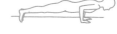

FOUR-LIMBED STAFF POSE
CHATURANGA DANDASANA
(chat-ur-ANGA don-DAH-sah-nah)

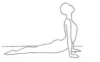

UPWARD-FACING DOG
URDHVA MUKHA SVANASANA
(OOrd-va MOO-ka svan-AH-sah-nah)

DOWNWARD-FACING DOG
ADHO MUKHA SVANASANA
(ODD-ho MOO-ka svan-AH-sah-nah)

Standing Poses

CHAIR POSE (or FIERCE POSE)
UTKATASANA
(OOT-kah-TAH-sah-nah)

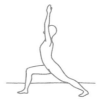

WARRIOR POSE I
VIRABHADRASANA I
(vee-rah-bah-DRAH-sah-nah)

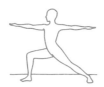

WARRIOR POSE II
VIRABHADRASANA II
(vee-rah-bah-DRAH-sah-nah)

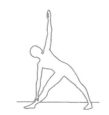

EXTENDED TRIANGLE POSE
UTTHITA TRIKONASANA
(oo-TEE-tah trik-cone-AH-sah-nah)

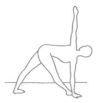

REVOLVED TRIANGLE POSE
PARIVRTTA TRIKONASANA
(pah-ree-VRIT-ah trik-cone-AH-sah-nah)

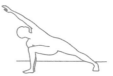

EXTENDED SIDE ANGLE POSE
UTTHITA PARSVAKONASANA
(oo-TEE-tah pars-vah-cone-AH-sah-nah)

Balancing Poses

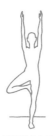

TREE POSE
VRKSASANA
(vrik-SHAHS-ah-nah)

DANCER'S POSE
NATARAJASANA
(nah-tah-rah-JAHS-ah-nah)

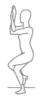

EAGLE POSE
GARUDASANA
(gah-roo-DAH-sah-nah)

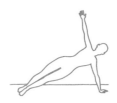

SIDE PLANK POSE
VASISTHASANA
(vah-see-STAHS-ah-nah)

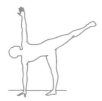

HALF MOON POSE
ARDHA CHANDRASANA
(ARE-duh chan-DRAH-sah-nah)

Seated Poses, Twists, and Abdominal Strengtheners

STAFF POSE
DANDASANA
(dahn-DAH-sah-nah)

BOUND ANGLE POSE
BADDHA KONASANA
(BAH-dah cone-AH-sah-nah)

COW-FACE POSE
GOMUKHASANA
(GO-moo-KAH-sah-nah)

SEATED TWIST

FULL BOAT POSE
PARIPURNA NAVASANA
(pah-ree-POOR-nah nah-VAH-sah-nah)

Forward Bends and Hip Openers

SEATED FORWARD BEND
PASCHIMOTTANASANA
(PAH-she-mow-tahn-AH-sah-nah)

SEATED WIDE-LEGGED FORWARD BEND
UPAVISTHA KONASANA
(ooh-pah-VEE-stah cone-AH-sah-nah)

HEAD-TO-KNEE POSE
JANU SIRSASANA
(JAH-new shear-SHAH-sah-nah)

PIGEON POSE

Backbends

LOCUST POSE

SALABHASANA

(sha-lah-BAHS-ah-nah)

COBRA POSE

BHUJANGASANA

(boo-jahng-AH-sah-nah)

BOW POSE

DHANURASANA

(dahn-your-AHS-ah-nah)

BRIDGE POSE

SETU BANDHA SARVANGASANA

(set-oo BAHN-dah sar-vahn-GAH-sah-nah)

CAMEL POSE

USTRASANA

(oo-STRAS-ah-nah)

FISH POSE

MATSYASANA

(mats-YAS-ah-nah)

Inversions

LEGS UP THE WALL
VIPARITA KARANI
(vi-pa-REE-ta ka-RON-ee)

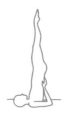

SHOULDER STAND
SARVANGASANA
(sar-van-GA-sah-nah)

Resting Poses

CHILD'S POSE
BALASANA
(bah-LAS-ah-nah)

CORPSE POSE
SAVASANA
(sha-VAS-ah-nah)

6ᵒᴰ   Gen 2/16 TD